Common Neurological Problems in General Paediatrics

Richard E Appleton MB BS DCH MA(Oxon) FRCP FRCPCH

Consultant Paediatric Neurologist and Honorary Clinical Lecturer in Child Health, The Roald Dahl EEG Unit, Alder Hey Children's Hospital, Liverpool, UK

AC Boudewyn Peters MD PhD

Professor of Child Neurology, Wilhelmina Children's Hospital, University Medical Center, Utrecht, The Netherlands

MARTIN DUNITZ

© 2003 Martin Dunitz Ltd, a member of the Taylor & Francis group

First published in the United Kingdom in 2003
by Martin Dunitz Ltd, Taylor & Francis Group plc, 11 New Fetter Lane, London EC4P 4EE

Tel.: +44 (0) 20 7482 2202
Fax.: +44 (0) 20 7267 0159
E-mail: info@dunitz.co.uk
Website: http://www.dunitz.co.uk

Although every effort has been made to ensure that all owners of copyright material have been acknowledged in this publication, we would be glad to acknowledge in subsequent reprints or editions any omissions brought to our attention.

The Author has asserted his right under the Copyright, Designs and Patents Act 1988 to be identified as the Author of this Work.

Although every effort has been made to ensure that drug doses and other information are presented accurately in this publication, the ultimate responsibility rests with the prescribing physician. Neither the publishers nor the authors can be held responsible for errors or for any consequences arising from the use of information contained herein. For detailed prescribing information or instructions on the use of any product or procedure discussed herein, please consult the prescribing information or instructional material issued by the manufacturer.

A CIP record for this book is available from the British Library.

ISBN 1-85317-736-9

Distributed in the USA by
Fulfilment Center
Taylor & Francis
7625 Empire Drive
Florence, KY 41042, USA
Toll Free Tel: +1 800 634 7064
E-mail: cserve@routledge_ny.com

Distributed in Canada by
Taylor & Francis
74 Rolark Drive
Scarborough, Ontario M1R 4G2, Canada
Toll Free Tel: +1 877 226 2237
E-mail: tal_fran@istar.ca

Distributed in the rest of the world by
Thomson Publishing Services Ltd.
Cheriton House
North Way
Andover, Hampshire SP10 5BE, UK
Tel:+44 (0)1264 332424
E-mail: salesorder.tandf@thomsonpublishingservices.co.uk

Composition by Wearset Ltd, Boldon, Tyne and Wear

Printed and bound in Great Britain by The Cromwell Press

Contents

Preface

Neurological symptoms account for at least one third of referrals to or consultations within a general paediatric outpatient department. These symptoms may range form the 'trivial' to the 'profound' and may reflect anything from parental or child anxiety to a severe and potentially progressive underlying disorder of the peripheral or central nervous system that may have important management and genetic implications.

The primary objective of this book is to provide a quick, logical and practical overview of some of the more common presenting neurological symptoms or signs manifest by children in general paediatric practice. The book emphasises the importance of the clinical approach to these children by providing a rational framework to a detailed assessment of each symptom, including a guide to the most relevant aspects of the history and examination and appropriate investigations, a brief outline of management and when to consider specialist advice.

It is not the purpose of this book to provide a comprehensive account of the specialism of paediatric neurology and its practice. Should the reader so wish, additional details and information on additional neurological symptoms and specific neurological disorders can be found in a number of the many excellent reference textbooks on paediatric neurology, epilepsy and neuromuscular disease.

The book is organised on the basis of patient presentation in the following four areas:
- The child with fits, faints and funny turns
- The child who is floppy
- The child with headaches
- The child with development delay/learning difficulties.

Acknowledgements

REA would like to dedicate this book to his teachers and mentors in Paediatric Neurology, in Vancouver, Canada (John Crichton, Henry Dunn, Kevin Farrell, Alan Hill and James Jan), Newcastle-upon-Tyne, UK (David Gardner-Medwin) and Paris, France (Jean Aicardi); thank you for your example, your enthusiasm and your support.

ACBP would like to dedicate this book to Mariet van der Schans, MD, librarian, willing to help throughout the years, and always in a friendly way. Thank you, Mariet! Also Richard Appleton, Oebo Brouwer, Wim Feikema, Aagje Jennekens and Joost Haan for their comments, positive criticism, enthusiasm and support.

Richard and Boudewyn would like to thank James Michael for permission to use one of his earlier photographs.

chapter 1

Fits, faints and funny turns

Introduction

It is likely that at least 25–30% of children referred to a paediatric clinic with the question 'is it epilepsy?' do **not** have epilepsy but are experiencing other types of paroxysmal events. An incorrect label of epilepsy can have unfortunate and serious consequences. The child may not only experience adverse side-effects from unnecessary medication but the 'stigma' of epilepsy will influence the child's daily and importantly, future life. A false-positive diagnosis is potentially far more harmful than a delay in the diagnosis of genuine epilepsy.

'Fits' or 'seizures' are by definition episodic, but not necessarily epileptic. They point to an episode of (transient) alteration of cerebral function, and further clarification is crucial. In particular in (very) young children the whole spectrum of 'fits, faints, and funny turns' may worry not only the parents but also the clinician faced with these episodes.

In this chapter efforts are made to enable the paediatrician to make **a positive diagnosis other than 'epilepsy'.** Although special emphasis is given to non-epileptic phenomena, a few sentences on making the diagnosis of epilepsy are unavoidable.

Table 1.1 provides an overview of the conditions described and discussed in this chapter.

Table1.1 Overview of fits, faints and funny turns (selected)

Group	Condition	Age	Diagnostic clues (history)	What may make you think of epilepsy?	page
Episodes associated with sleep	Benign, neonatal sleep myoclonus	<1 year	never involves the face; never wakens the child from sleep	(migrating) myoclonic seizures	7
	parasomnias	<6 years	first hours of sleep, no memory; one episode a night	behaviour during nocturnal frontal epileptic seizures	
Episodes associated with feeding	gastro-esophageal reflux (Sandifer syndrome)	up to 6 years	after feeding; failure to thrive; pH monitoring	'tonic fits'	8
Syncope or anoxic seizures	apnoea during crying ('blue breath-holding')	first months of life – 5 years	always a provoking stimulus; crying	tonic/opisthotonic posturing, even with jerks	11–12
	reflex anoxic seizure	up to 6 years if not older	always some provocation; crying brief or absent	unconsciousness, with stiffening and jerks = tonic–clonic seizure	12–13

Group	Condition	Age	Diagnostic clues (history)	What may make you think of epilepsy?	page
	vasovagal syncope	all ages (but usually older children)	stimuli (obvious or subtle); specific situations; presyncopal feeling	unconsciousness of longer duration, with jerks or even a brief tonic phase	13–14
	long QT-syndrome	all ages (but usually older children)	anoxic seizure or syncope during exercise, sleep or specific stimuli (e.g. sudden shock or pain)	see reflex anoxic seizures	14–15
Paroxysmal movement disorders	self-gratification, masturbation	first months of life – 4 years (or older)	stimulation-seeking; at times of stress or boredom; episodes can be interrupted	frequently rhythmic movements; grunts; 'trance'	15–16
	shuddering spells	<5 years	'as if cold water was poured down the child's back'	short myoclonic or clonic seizures	17
	hyperekplexia	from birth throughout life	family history; stiffening on handling	startle epilepsy; myoclonic seizures	17
	benign paroxysmal vertigo	<5 years	family history; migraine	atonic or complex partial seizures	17

Table1.1 Overview of fits, faints and funny turns (selected) (*continued*)

Group	Condition	Age	Diagnostic clues (history)	What may make you think of epilepsy?	page
	paroxysmal dyskinesias	all ages	often induced by movements	episodes may be very brief and respond to anti-epileptic medication	18–19
	stereotypies	all ages	mentally handicapped children	staring, rhythmic movements, tonic posturing also genuine epilepsy	19–20
Behavioural and psychogenic disorders	psychogenic non-epileptic seizures	>5 years	the place or setting in which they occur; teenage girls; video, video-EEG monitoring	child often (but not always) also has genuine epilepsy	20–21

The approach to paroxysmal episodes

- Recurrent, paroxysmal episodes
  ⇓
- History taking (time must be taken to obtain a detailed history of the beginning, middle and end of the episode).
  ⇓
- Ask for eyewitnesses, call the schoolteacher, and any other relevant people who may have **seen** the episodes.
  ⇓

The first episode
(if appropriate: detailed questioning on the first episode)
Further episodes
(new details, differences from first episode; time between first and further episodes)
  ⇓

The setting	Where: at home, at school, in bed, elsewhere. What was the child doing: awake, asleep; active, at rest; alone, in company; watching TV, playing on the computer; other obvious provocation or trigger.
The beginning	Any feelings before the episode started. What was the first thing that was seen to be different. What happened next, and next, and next . . .
The middle	Alert, impairment or loss of consciousness;

The middle (continued):
- do not accept terms such as; 'not well', or 'not being there'.

Movements; limbs, right-left, face; rhythmic, non-rhythmic;
- do not simply accept words like 'fit', 'shaking', 'twitching', 'jerking';
- let parents/eyewitnesses demonstrate or mime the movements or do them yourself and ask 'were the movements like this or like that . . . '

Tone; increased, decreased; loss of body tone.
Any other features: colour change; urinary or faecal incontinence; tongue-biting, etc . . .

The end   How did the episode stop: was it gradual or abrupt.
           What was the child like afterwards: confused, sleepy,
           alert. When was the child completely back to normal.

- Family, medical history

⇓

first decision

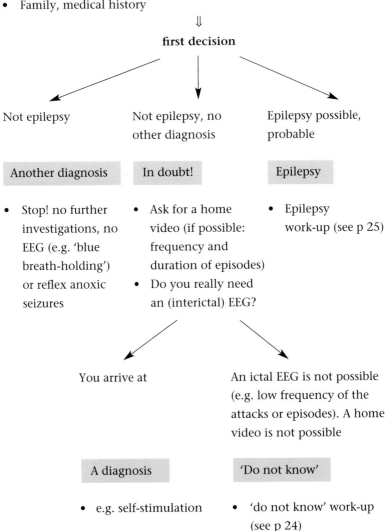

Not epilepsy   Not epilepsy, no   Epilepsy possible,
                other diagnosis   probable

Another diagnosis   In doubt!   Epilepsy

- Stop! no further   • Ask for a home   • Epilepsy
  investigations, no   video (if possible: work-up (see p 25)
  EEG (e.g. 'blue   frequency and
  breath-holding')   duration of episodes)
  or reflex anoxic   • Do you really need
  seizures   an (interictal) EEG?

You arrive at   An ictal EEG is not possible
                                 (e.g. low frequency of the
                                 attacks or episodes). A home
                                 video is not possible

A diagnosis   'Do not know'

- e.g. self-stimulation   • 'do not know' work-up
                                   (see p 24)

Episodes associated with sleep

Benign sleep myoclonus is characterized by myoclonic jerks occurring only during sleep **(in all sleep states)**, in particular starting in the first month of life. As the jerking may migrate from one limb to the other or show a more or less rhythmic aspect, the possibility of 'epilepsy' may arise. In addition, the duration (sometimes more than 30 minutes, of varying intensity) and clustering of these movements can be confusing. Waking the children results in an acute interruption of the myoclonic movements. Jerking is never seen in the alert state. Other clues are: no jerks are seen in the face or eyes, and the jerks do not wake the infant. Benign sleep myoclonus occurs particularly in the first month of life but can be seen throughout the first year of life.

The normal jerks (hypnagogic) that occur on **falling asleep** are different. They disappear in the deeper sleep states and may occur at all ages.

Nocturnal disturbances of behaviour are common in children. Episodic types of behaviour occurring exclusively during **sleep (parasomnias)** may be of epileptic origin, but are more often not. Night terrors, sleep walking, violently turning over, sitting up, muttering, moaning, vocalizations and similar features are so called **arousal disorders**. They occur in the first two or three hours of sleep (deep non-REM sleep) and the child has no memory of the episode the next morning.

Nocturnal epileptic (complex partial) seizures may have symptoms overlapping non-epileptic parasomnias such as complicated, sometimes bizarre automatisms and vocalizations. Nocturnal complex partial (mostly frontal or temporal) seizures typically occur frequently (sometimes multiple episodes each night), show very stereotyped behaviour, including posturing, grunting and swallowing, and have an abrupt onset and termination. These children also usually, but not always, have more typical daytime epileptic seizures.

Episodes associated with feeding

In the **very young** (e.g. first 3 months of life), paroxysmal events **during feeding** such as episodes of sudden motionless stare, sudden involuntary movements or changes in tone, 'abnormal' roving eye movements, or cessation of breathing are very common. These episodes, which defy precise classification, are usually harmless and transient.

Episodic events that occur not during, but **after feeding** (occurrence within minutes to an hour) may be due to **gastro-oesophageal reflux (GER)**. In these cases, there may be a history of prior regurgitation, recurrent vomiting or spitting up, rumination, failure to thrive, irritability during feeding and episodes of aspiration (coughing during or after feeding).

Episodes of body posturing, e.g. stiffening, opisthotonus, dystonia or torticollis may be associated with GER and may initially be misdiagnosed as tonic seizures or paroxysmal dystonia. This posturing is often called **Sandifer syndrome** (Figure 1.1), and is believed to represent a response that relieves the discomfort associated with GER. This is difficult to understand since the complex contortions often promote GER. The relationship between symptoms and positional changes is not always clear. Some children reflux more in the upright than in the supine position and parents' comments are often very helpful. In general children are more likely to reflux while awake than while asleep. GER is common in children with other disorders, in particular with (severe) mental handicap, and is often accompanied by episodes of aspiration. The diagnosis of Sandifer syndrome is often delayed, in particular in the retarded child who also has epilepsy – with the posturing being ascribed to 'tonic epileptic fits'. In particular the absence of vomiting may be a pitfall. Oesophageal pH monitoring with values <4 is diagnostic and video-fluoroscopy will usually confirm aspiration.

GER is common in infants, but **GER-associated obstructive apnoea** is rare. The key features are apnoea while awake, feeding within the previous hour, sudden staring or startled appearance, rigid postures followed by hypotonia, and absence of coughing, gagging or choking. Change in skin colour (flushed red to pallor and cyanosis) may be seen. An episode

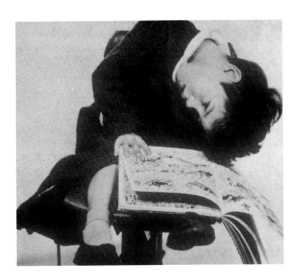

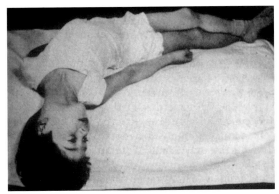

Figure 1.1 *Four-year-old boy with Sandifer's syndrome due to hiatus hernia and associated gastro-oesophageal reflux: (a) posture usually adopted for reading and (b) posture usually adopted when lying down. (Reproduced from Kinsbourne M. Lancet 1964; 6: 1058–61 with permission from Elsevier Science Ltd.)*

of apnoea is commonly provoked by a nappy change (flexion of legs) or change from lying to a seated position. Episodes of airway obstruction at the time of GER have been demonstrated.

Gastro-oesophageal reflux should be kept in mind in every child presenting with an Apparent Life Threatening Event (**ALTE**). In particular, during sleep these children have GER, possibly with reflux-induced hypoxemia.

Syncopes or anoxic seizures

Definition, terminology, features

Clinical definition of syncope: an abrupt, transient loss of consciousness and change in postural tone with no clearly identified aetiology at the time of presentation

Syncope is a very common, paroxysmal disorder, and affects all age groups in childhood and beyond. It is, however, an umbrella term and needs clarification.

The clinical symptomology of syncope (Greek: 'cutting off') is based on a sudden reduction in cerebral perfusion by oxygenated blood (cerebral hypoxaemia). Essentially, a reduction of cerebral blood flow itself (e.g. asystole) or a fall in oxygen content (e.g. suffocation) or a combination of the two are the underlying mechanisms.

The duration of unconsciousness and the degree of other clinical features depend on the mechanisms of the syncope and on the age of the child. The symptomatology in children has been studied systematically during the ocular compression test (Figure 1.2) and the head-up tilt test.

The terminology is often confusing. Syncope and anoxic seizure are often interchangeable.

Features observed in anoxic seizures. or: why anoxic seizures are confused with epileptic seizures

- unconsciousness
- atonia (complete loss of tone)
- tonic stiffening
    opisthotonus

flexion of upper limbs
- jerks [either isolated (myoclonic) or repeated, briefly (clonic)]
- eye jerks and deviation; head turning
- snort
- disorientation; agitation; postictal sleep
- urinary incontinence
- autonomic phenomena (salivation, cyanosis, pallor, flush)

Blue breath-holding spells

These are well known and assumed to be benign. An obvious provocation such as pain, frustration, or fear is crucial in establishing the

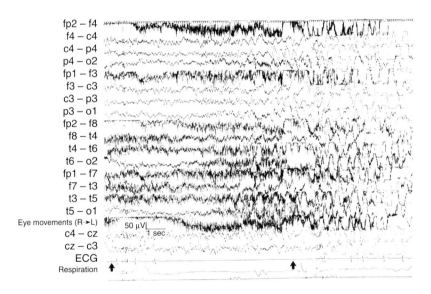

Figure 1.2 *Five-year-old boy with a history of reflex anoxic seizures, undergoing ocular compression during simultaneous EEG and ECG recordings. Arrows indicate start and finish of ocular (eyeball) pressure for a period of 10 seconds. ECG demonstrates a period of asystole for 8 seconds and 3 seconds after the onset of asystole, the EEG shows only diffuse slowing. During this period the boy demonstrated tonic posturing of all four limbs, described by his mother as 'the fit'.*

diagnosis. The child begins to cry, which may either be restricted to two or three cries or whining, broken sounds, or a prolonged, gradually intensifying scream. Then, the child reaches a point of noiselessness, the mouth is open, the breath is held in full expiration ('breath holding'), and 'an ominous silence accompanies the period of apnoea'. The lips and even the face turn bluish, but then, with a laboured inspiration followed by crying, the spell resolves itself. There is only a very brief or no obvious loss of consciousness.

However, if 'breath-holding' continues, cyanosis deepens, the child loses consciousness, and a change in postural tone is observed, limpness rapidly changing to a tonic/opisthotonic posture. Occasionally, body jerks and urinary incontinence are observed. The child may appear drowsy and exhausted, but within several minutes the majority of children are alert and active and only a minority are sleepy and inactive for an hour or two.

Although the time of onset is most commonly within the first one and a half years, the episodes may start in the first weeks of life.

Pallid breath-holding (pallid infantile syncope, pallid syncopal attack, reflex anoxic seizure, cardiovagal syncope)

Pallid or white breath-holding spells, as opposed to blue breath-holding, is an inappropriate term as we are not dealing with breath-holding. Here, a vagal-mediated cardioinhibitory mechanism is activated. We prefer the term **reflex anoxic seizure** or **pallid syncopal attack**.

The history is again crucial – there is always a history of a painful or emotional stimulus such as a head bump (usually on the back of the head), a fall, pain or sudden fright followed by crying and then, within a few seconds, by going limp, lying deathly still with eyes fixed upwards, and abruptly stiffening with an arched back and hands fisted. Within 10–30 seconds the child relaxes, opens its eyes and responds. The child's face is very pale or even white.

If the history is obvious, an ocular compression test to try and reproduce the episodes is unnecessary.

Importantly, the painful trigger or sudden fright may not have been observed at all, or not on every occasion. If an obvious stimulus has been observed at least in a few episodes, and the paroxysms are more or less uniform, the diagnosis of reflex anoxic seizures would appear to be correct. However, without any historical evidence of any painful or frightening stimulus, the diagnosis must be seriously questioned. A second important point is that the duration of the episodes may be quite long: the period of cerebral hypoxia and unconsciousness can last for many minutes and the clinical features are not limited to stiffening, but 'jerks', 'spasms', urinary incontinence and disorientation or confusion after the episode may be described by the parents. All these phenomena may suggest an epileptic seizure – which again emphasizes the point about asking if anything painful happened to the child first before the attack.

Diagnostically the most important syncope not to be confused with a reflex anoxic seizure is the **long QT syndrome** (see p 14), or some other cardiac arrhythmia. A positive family history (including sudden deaths), syncopes without warning or syncopes occurring during exercise, sleep or after a sudden loud noise (even an alarm clock!) should raise strong suspicion of an underlying cardiac arrhythmia and necessitate a paediatric cardiology consultation.

Breath-holding: mixed type

It is unusual for breath-holding spells (cyanotic) and reflex anoxic seizures (pallid) to occur in the same child (i.e. syncopes of respiratory and cardiogenic origin, respectively, on separate occasions). However, there is a mixed type of breath-holding in which expiratory apnoea and bradycardia or asystole both play a role. In practice this may result in children who not only turn bluish, but also show the whole range of features seen in reflex anoxic seizures.

Vasovagal syncope (neurocardiogenic = neurally mediated hypotension or bradycardia; vasodepressor syncope, fainting)

The pathophysiology of vasovagal syncopes is complicated. In classical 'fainting' after a trigger, heart rate and muscle blood flow initially increase, followed by a sudden drop in heart rate and hypotension, resulting in the faint. However, as both cardioinhibitory and vasodepressor mechanisms may be active, clinical symptomatology may result in diagnostic errors. In particular, the convulsive syncopes may be confused with epileptic seizures.

The term 'fainting' is used in older children, and is – incorrectly – restricted to symptoms starting in an upright position.

Again, history of (subtle) stimuli and the specific situations in which the episodes occur are important in establishing a correct diagnosis. A positive family history for fainting, going limp, having 'fits' or 'black-outs' is commonly found. Stimuli are highly different, e.g. bathing (supine!), hair combing/brushing (pain as comb or brush catching in and pulling or tearing the hair), venepuncture (supine!). Important, pre-syncopal features include dizziness, greying out of vision, voices and noises sounding distant, tinnitus, abdominal pain, feeling cold and clammy – all present before a **gradual** loss of consciousness.

In infants or young children not able to describe these pre-syncopal features, diagnostic confusion with epilepsy is based on the following symptoms:

a) onset of unconsciousness is abrupt;
b) duration of unconsciousness is more than one minute;
c) jerks or convulsions, or even a tonic–clonic phase, are observed;
d) abdominal pain (as a pre-syncopal symptom) is interpreted as an epigastric aura. An aura and a convulsive syncope are mistaken for an epileptic seizure;
e) incontinence is present;
f) frequency is high.

All of the above features may all be seen during vasovagal syncopes, and a few 'jerks' or 'twitches' may be seen in at least 80% of cases!

Cardiac disorders and anoxic seizures

Cardiac arrhythmias may result in a simple or convulsive syncope or an anoxic seizure.

Congenital **long QT syndrome (LQTS)** is characterized by QT-interval prolongation on the ECG and polymorphic ventricular arrhythmias (torsade de pointes) that may lead to syncope and sudden cardiac death. There is a classic subdivision of LQTS into Romano–Ward syndrome (usually autosomal dominant inheritance) and Jervell and Lange-Nielsen syndrome (inherited as an autosomal recessive trait and associated with congenital deafness).

Key points associated with LQTS

- Syncopes or seizures during exercise, sporting activity (in particular swimming or diving), auditory stimuli, startle (e.g. from a sudden loud noise or an alarm clock when asleep), emotional stress or shock, or associated with sleep.
- Family history of syncopes, seizures, or sudden death under age 50; congenital deafness (sensorineural).

A routine ECG may **not** adequately exclude LQTS and referral to a paediatric cardiologist **must** be undertaken if there is a possibility that the child may have LQTS. The disorder is potentially fatal but, importantly, is treatable.

Other cardiac arrhythmias or congenital (corrected) cardiac defects leading to anoxic seizures or syncopes are usually not a diagnostic problem.

Paroxysmal movement disorders (with or without impaired consciousness)

Self-stimulation, masturbation

Many physicians seem to be unfamiliar with normal infantile sexual development. The parents' description of the child's behaviour is interpreted as an epileptic phenomenon or abdominal discomfort, resulting in a number of unnecessary investigations and even drug treatments.

Characteristic features of self-gratification and masturbation (Figure 1.3):

- adduction and tightening of the legs
- rhythmic pelvic movements
- staring, absent-minded, 'trance-like'
- sweating and facial flushing
- grunting noises
- the child can usually be interrupted or distracted from these movements

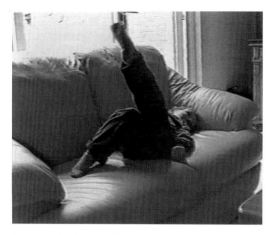

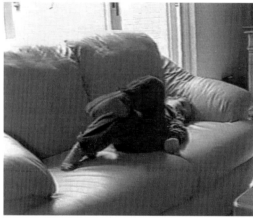

Figure 1.3 *Four and a half-year-old boy with frequent episodes of self-stimulation, during which he would demonstrate non-rhythmic movements of his left leg with adduction of both upper legs, slight facial-flushing and intact consciousness. Most occurred when he was watching children's programmes on the television.*

A videotape of the episodes taken at home or at school is usually diagnostic!

Masturbation in public is part of normal sexual development in young children. In general, an explanation of this behaviour is usually sufficient to reassure the parents and, importantly, the occurrence of these episodes in public usually resolves before the age of seven or eight years. The frequency of masturbation in the very young often increases in situations of emotional deprivation, family stresses or sexual abuse. The physician should keep this in mind when self-gratification persists in public.

'Shuddering spells' in infancy or early childhood

Shivering or 'shuddering' movements for several seconds without impairment of consciousness, occurring daily, in otherwise normal children, sometimes at times of excitement. A good description is 'as if cold water was poured down the child's back!'

The condition is benign, transient and may be related to benign myoclonus of early infancy. There is sometimes a family history of benign essential tremor in these children.

Startle disease, hyperekplexia

This is a very rare, hereditary disorder (channelopathy) that may be inherited in an autosomal dominant or recessive pattern; the gene defect is on chromosome 5q. In the dominant form, the condition is relatively easy to recognize in the young child. Exaggerated startle reflexes to unexpected, particularly auditory and tactile, stimuli are characteristic. The characteristic startle response is often elicited easily by tapping the infant's nose – the 'normal' infant will startle two or three times but in the infant with hyperekplexia the startle response will continue each time that the nose is tapped. In addition, the baby stiffens on handling, e.g. changing a diaper or bathing. At rest the infant's tone normalizes. This stiffness normalizes during the first years of life. In the minor form, symptoms are restricted to excessive startle reactions without stiffness. It is **not** startle epilepsy. Clonazepam is often very helpful, but the condition may persist well into adult life. One form of hyperekplexia may be associated with epilepsy and is more difficult to treat.

Benign paroxysmal vertigo (BPV)

This comprises of sudden, brief attacks during which the child falls, without impairment of consciousness, usually accompanied by pallor or vomiting, and, if closely observed, nystagmus. The older child complains of dizziness during the attack. These children frequently develop migraine, and there is often a family history of migraine. However, the relationship between the so-called 'migraine equivalents' (of which BPV may be one type) and migraine later in childhood is inconstant and even debatable.

Episodic ataxia

There are many episodic ataxias, a number of which are familial and may have an onset in childhood. Attacks may last seconds to minutes and are comprised of loss of balance, sometimes provoked by startle and exercise. Muscle twitches (myokymia) between attacks may be seen. Disorders of both calcium and potassium channels have been described, and some may be respond to acetazolamide.

Paroxysmal dyskinesias

One of the most common types is a dystonia, accompanied by choreoathetosis, which may be induced by movement (kinesigenic) lasting some minutes, and without any alteration in consciousness. It may occur sporadically or in families (autosomal dominant inheritance). Although not of epileptic origin this rare disorder may respond to low-dose anti-epileptic medication, specifically carbamazepine, lamotrigine or phenytoin. This group of conditions probably represents one or more channelopathies.

Tics, paroxysmal torticollis, paroxysmal tonic up-gaze, spasmus nutans

The nonrhythmic nature of tics or tic disorders is obvious, and diagnosis should not be difficult. The stereotyped, repetitive movements are irregular. The most common simple tics are motor and include eyeblinking, head turning or facial twitches (occasionally misdiagnosed as 'focal fits' or myoclonus). Tics may evolve to more complicated movements, and if accompanied by sniffing, grunting, snorting or vocalization, are more appropriately termed Gilles de la Tourette syndrome. These children usually have attentional deficits, mild learning difficulties (which antedate the tic disorder) and features of obsessive–compulsive disorder. Simple motor tics should be best ignored (when they will tend to resolve spontaneously), but if they become intrusive or develop into the Tourette syndrome, then drug treatment may be necessary (e.g. haloperidol, pimozide, clonidine), as well as involving child psychology/psychiatry.

Paroxysmal torticollis is characterized by recurrent episodes of an abnormal rotation and inclination of the head on one side. An episode may last from minutes to days. The shorter the episode, the greater is the risk of misdiagnosing epilepsy. There is a possible relationship with the later development of childhood migraine. The disorder is usually self-limited. Acute and persistent torticollis (i.e. a persistent head tilt) should raise the possibility of a lesion in the posterior fossa or paresis of the fourth cranial nerve.

Paroxysmal tonic up-gaze is a rare syndrome, described mainly in infants, of sudden, persistent (seconds) upturning ('rolling up') of the eyeballs. Potentially misleading features include 'collapse-like' episodes in some patients. Symptoms gradually resolve between three and four years of age. The precise cause of these episodes is unknown.

Spasmus nutans consists of a triad: nystagmus, head nodding and a head tilt. The nystagmoid movements may be more obvious in one eye. Rarely, some confusion with 'epileptic seizures' may arise as symptoms may fluctuate during the day. The condition is benign although rarely it may be due to a space-occupying lesion (e.g. optic glioma or arachnoid/ porencephalic cyst).

Benign non-epileptic infantile spasms

Serial jerks or flexion spasms occurring in the first year of life will usually raise the suspicion of infantile spasms. However, the EEG is normal during both wakefulness and sleep and also during a 'spasm'. In addition, the child's development progresses normally. The spasms cannot be differentiated clinically from the infantile spasms seen in West syndrome. However, treatment of the benign, non-epileptic spasms is unnecessary, the prognosis is excellent and the spasms resolve before two years of age.

Stereotyped, repetitive episodes in the mentally handicapped child

In the neurologically impaired child it may be difficult to differentiate abnormal, stereotyped, repetitive episodes from epileptic seizures. These non-epileptic, stereotyped episodes (stereotypies) tend to be particularly common when the child is either excited or upset. Many of these children also have definite epilepsy, and show interictal abnormal (including spike or spike and slow wave) activity on their EEG. Video-EEG monitoring may be necessary to accurately diagnose these episodes. It is very important to differentiate these non-epileptic, stereotyped movements from the genuine seizures (including non-convulsive status epilepticus) to avoid over-treatment with anti-epileptic drugs and prevent drug toxicity.

Stereotyped behaviours mistaken for epileptic seizures in children with (severe) mental handicap
- staring
- rhythmic movements (body rocking, head shaking or nodding, arm or hand flapping or clapping)
- abnormal eye movements, including sustained eye deviation
- repetitive mouth movements (chewing, tongue thrusting)
- tonic posturing
- episodic hyperventilation with or without rhythmic movements
- tremor

Behavioural and psychogenic disorders

Psychogenic non-epileptic seizures (PNES) (non-epileptic attack disorder, pseudo-seizures, pseudo-epileptic seizures)

This condition describes episodic behaviour that resembles an epileptic seizure, but is not associated with EEG abnormalities. Even experienced observers may have difficulties in differentiating a psychogenic non-epileptic seizure, particularly if the child also has genuine epileptic seizures. These children usually model their non-epileptic events on their epileptic seizures, including tonic–clonic seizures. In children who do not know what epileptic seizures look like, their events usually take the form of swoons and prolonged blank spells (staring), or occasionally, single or repeated twitches of an arm or leg or thrashing of the whole body.

Implicit in the definition of PNES is the idea that individuals do not consciously produce or control their (non-epileptic) events, and thus are not malingerers. The diagnosis is important, not only for unnecessary medical treatment, but also to search for (and hopefully find and treat) underlying causes, such as anxiety, dysfunctional (family) relationships, history of physical/sexual abuse or neglect, or attention-seeking behaviour. Management intervention by a child psychiatrist or clinical psychologist is frequently successful.

Video-EEG monitoring may be extremely helpful in the diagnosis of bizarre and persistent PNES. There are a number of features that are helpful in differentiating epileptic versus non-epileptic attacks (Table 1.2). Psychogenic non-epileptic attacks rarely occur in:

- children under the age of six or seven years;
- boys under the age of 10 years;
- sleep, or on waking. Episodes that are 'bizarre' and occur either during sleep or on waking from sleep will usually be epileptic – particularly complex partial epileptic seizures, and usually arising from the frontal rather than the temporal lobes;
- places or situations where there is no one else to witness them.

Miscellaneous

Infancy: episodes associated with vaccination

Collapse after pertussis vaccine, in particular after a first vaccination, is very frightening to parents and occurs in approximately 1 in 2000 doses (usually only after the first vaccination). This hypotonic–hyporesponsive episode or shock-like syndrome presents within 12 hours after vaccination with sudden loss of muscle tone, pallor and unresponsiveness, with full recovery within minutes to an hour. The cause is unknown, but may be related to a vaso-vagal (syncopal) mechanism.

Such a reaction following pertussis vaccination does not constitute a

Table1.2 Epileptic seizures versus psychogenic non-epileptic seizures

	Epileptic seizure	*Psychogenic non-epileptic seizure*
aura	may be present, of relatively long duration (>10 seconds)	if present, of very short duration (1–5 seconds)
movements	more stereotyped clonic jerks: flexor, rhythmic; all extremities involved; waning of movements	less stereotyped; sudden onset and offset; bilateral, flexor and extensor out of phase in involved limbs; violent, asynchronous flailing of limbs; unusual movements e.g. pelvic thrusting
consciousness	typically either lost or impaired	unimpaired but may appear to be unresponsive, even to painful stimuli; active resistance to eye opening
automatisms	simple (lip smacking, picking at clothes); complex (dressing/ undressing, walking)	may be bizarre
language	initial scream, groans, mumbling	swearing, yelling; vulgarities; groaning (which usually varies if spoken to or stimulated)
behaviour	not combative	combative, bizarre
Incontinence	frequent	rare
self-injury	tongue biting frequent (side of tongue); friction (carpet) burns	rare (tip of tongue)
post-ictal	confusion, headache, drowsiness	rare
frequency	usually single episodes	may continue, cluster-like
ictal-EEG	epileptiform (rarely, EEG normal in deep, medial frontal lobe foci)	no specific abnormalities
witnesses	may be not present	almost always present
age	all ages	≥6 years

contraindication to continuing with the remainder of the child's vaccination schedule.

Munchausen syndrome by proxy

In Munchausen syndrome by proxy a parent (commonly the child's mother) falsifies and fabricates the illness of their children. Seizures and syncopes are a common symptom or presentation of this syndrome. As a consequence, nursing and medical staff are often persuaded to undertake extensive and sometimes invasive investigations. Medication, including anti-epileptic medication, may be inappropriately prescribed, which may cause further confusion by inducing side-effects that could be misdiagnosed as a different type of epileptic seizure or even an underlying and progressive neurological disorder.

In Munchausen syndrome, the child is abused by the actions of the perpetrator and may be compounded by the doctors who do not recognize this syndrome at an early stage. The parental actions may include either poisoning the child with excessive doses of prescribed drugs (including anti-epileptic drugs), salt (leading to hypernatraemic-induced seizures) or suffocating their child (leading to anoxia-induced seizures). The management of these families may be difficult but must be undertaken thoroughly to prevent further injury to the child – including even death.

Daydreaming

Daydreaming or 'not being there' is very commonly mistaken for absence epilepsy. During 'daydreaming' responsiveness to touch or blowing gently on the child's face is preserved and the child will usually respond immediately. Play, actions and speech will not be interrupted in mid-action or mid-sentence. School teachers are often the first people to 'identify' daydreaming, in particular in children with attention deficit hyperactivity disorder (ADHD), and may misinterpret them as absence seizures. Simple 'daydreaming' is particularly common in children when they are tired and are also watching television at the same time, or when they are bored – and this includes in the school classroom!

Narcolepsy

Irresistible onset of daytime sleepiness at any time and in any place is very rare in children, but may occur, even as young as two years of age. The accompanying cataplexy (loss of muscle tone on emotional provocation, e.g. laughter, sudden shock or fright) and hypnagogic hallucinations are even more rare. The EEG may be helpful – children with narcolepsy will, as soon as they fall asleep, enter deep sleep immediately without first going through the lighter stages of sleep.

'Do not know'

In the very young infant or child, many paroxysmal episodes are **not classifiable** either when first seen or even after further clinic visits. Additionally, many just resolve, without having been definitively diagnosed.

What to do with 'the unclassifiable episodes'?
Episodes that are **not** alarming (to parents, to the general practitioner, to the physician); infrequent episodes
- wait and see;
- routine follow-up is probably necessary, in case of the following: changes in pattern, frequency; restart diagnostic investigations.

Episodes that **are** alarming (duration, physical injury, place where it happens); very frequent episodes
- second opinion (e.g. paediatric neurologist).
- video-EEG monitoring;

A 'trial of medication' – specifically anti-epileptic medication – is **never** indicated.

Epilepsy

Urinary incontinence, stiffness, jerking and even alteration of consciousness may occur in many types of non-epileptic seizures. After
classifying a seizure as definitely epileptic, it is important to classify
the type of the seizures, the type of epilepsy (i.e. the epilepsy syndrome)
and the possible aetiology (idiopathic or symptomatic) (see further
reading).

Remember:

- more children have spikes, sharp waves or slow waves in their EEG
  who do not have epilepsy than those who do;
- it is 'preferable' to initially miss a correct diagnosis of epilepsy in a
  child, rather than inappropriately treat many children with drugs
  whose paroxysmal attacks or seizures are not epileptic;
- if in doubt about the nature and cause of a child's 'funny turns' or
  paroxysmal attacks, always ask for the opinion of an expert – a paediatric neurologist;
- never use a 'trial of medication' to try and prove or disprove a diagnosis of either epilepsy or another paroxysmal non-epileptic disorder.
  Up to 30% of children with genuine epilepsy will not have their
  seizures controlled by an anti-epileptic drug, so the lack of a child's
  response to an anti-epileptic drug does not necessarily prove that the
  child's episodes are not epileptic in origin.

Common pitfalls

The following non-epileptic paroxysms are most frequently confused
with 'epileptic seizures':

- episodes associated with sleep
- syncopes or anoxic seizures
- self-gratification (masturbation)
- stereotypies in the mentally handicapped child

Also:

- never use a 'trial of anti-epileptic medication' in 'do not know' cases
- always ask for specialist advice in 'do not know' situations.

Further reading

Appleton R, Gibbs J, Epilepsy in childhood and adolescence. Second edition. Martin Dunitz, London. 1998.

Daley HM, Appleton RE. Fits, faints and funny turns. Current Paediatrics 2000; 10: 22–7.

Donat JF, Wright FS. Episodic symptoms mistaken for seizures in the neurologically impaired child. Neurology 1990; 40: 156–57.

Irwin K, Edwards M, Robinson R. Psychogenic non-epileptic seizures: management and prognosis. Arch Dis Child 2000; 82: 474–78.

Maydell BV, Berenson F, Rothner D et al. Benign myoclonus of early infancy: an imitator of West's syndrome. J Child Neurol 2001; 16: 109–12.

McHarg ML, Shinnar S, Rascoff H, Walsh CA. Syncope in childhood. Pediatr Cardiol 1997; 18: 367–71.

Prensky AL. An approach to the child with paroxysmal phenomenon with emphasis on nonepileptic disorders. In: Dodson WE, Pellock JM (eds). Pediatric epilepsy: diagnosis and therapy. New York: Demos Publications, 1993. pp 63–80.

Stephenson JBP. Nonepileptic seizures, anoxic-epileptic seizures, and epileptic anoxic seizures. In: Wallace S (ed). Epilepsy in children. London: Chapman and Hall, 1996. pp 5–25.

chapter 2

The floppy infant

Introduction

The floppy infant is a common presentation or problem in paediatric practice and may be seen in a wide range of situations, most but not all due an underlying neurological disorder.

The primary objective of this chapter is to consider the child who has an abnormally low muscle tone (hypotonia). These infants may show different types or patterns of presentation in the first two years of life. Parents frequently complain that their child:

- is 'floppy';
- does not move much;
- lies in strange or odd positions;
- appears to have loose joints;
- is slow in learning or developing new skills – 'she won't hold her head up';
- is very easy to dress and undress – 'he just lies there'.

The floppy infant syndrome simply describes a symptom; it is not a specific syndrome and may be due to a wide range of underlying causes, including (Figure 2.1):

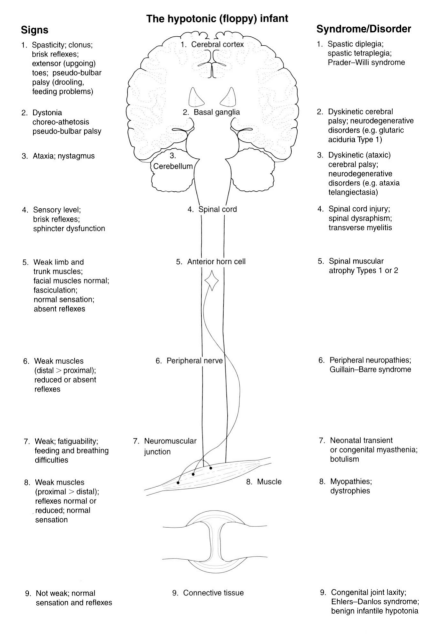

The hypotonic (floppy) infant

Signs		Syndrome/Disorder
1. Spasticity; clonus; brisk reflexes; extensor (upgoing) toes; pseudo-bulbar palsy (drooling, feeding problems)	1. Cerebral cortex	1. Spastic diplegia; spastic tetraplegia; Prader–Willi syndrome
2. Dystonia choreo-athetosis pseudo-bulbar palsy	2. Basal ganglia	2. Dyskinetic cerebral palsy; neurodegenerative disorders (e.g. glutaric aciduria Type 1)
3. Ataxia; nystagmus	3. Cerebellum	3. Dyskinetic (ataxic) cerebral palsy; neurodegenerative disorders (e.g. ataxia telangiectasia)
4. Sensory level; brisk reflexes; sphincter dysfunction	4. Spinal cord	4. Spinal cord injury; spinal dysraphism; transverse myelitis
5. Weak limb and trunk muscles; facial muscles normal; fasciculation; normal sensation; absent reflexes	5. Anterior horn cell	5. Spinal muscular atrophy Types 1 or 2
6. Weak muscles (distal > proximal); reduced or absent reflexes	6. Peripheral nerve	6. Peripheral neuropathies; Guillain–Barre syndrome
7. Weak; fatiguability; feeding and breathing difficulties	7. Neuromuscular junction	7. Neonatal transient or congenital myasthenia; botulism
8. Weak muscles (proximal > distal); reflexes normal or reduced; normal sensation	8. Muscle	8. Myopathies; dystrophies
9. Not weak; normal sensation and reflexes	9. Connective tissue	9. Congenital joint laxity; Ehlers–Danlos syndrome; benign infantile hypotonia

Figure 2.1 *Graphic illustration of possible causes of 'hypotonia' or 'the floppy infant' at different levels within the central nervous, peripheral nervous and musculoskeletal systems.*

- any temporary febrile or afebrile illness (any sick child may appear to be hypotonic);
- a systemic illness (e.g. cardiac, renal or hepatic failure);
- chromosomal abnormality (e.g. Down's syndrome);
- genetic syndrome (e.g. Prader–Willi syndrome);
- central (i.e. cerebral cortex, basal ganglia, cerebellar or spinal) nervous system disorder;
- neuromuscular disorder (i.e. peripheral neuropathy; neuromuscular junction defect; muscular dystrophy);
- connective tissue disorder (e.g. Ehlers-Danlos syndrome, congenital ligamentous laxity);
- metabolic or biochemical disorder (e.g. hypothyroidism or an organic acidaemia).

Approximately 80–90% of children who demonstrate hypotonia in the first year of life will be found to have a disorder of the central nervous system or a genetic/chromosomal disorder. The remaining 10–20% will have a peripheral neuromuscular or unidentified condition.

The most common peripheral (neuromuscular) causes of a hypotonic and weak infant presenting in the first year of life include:

- spinal muscular atrophy (specifically, Type 1 (severe Werdnig–Hoffman disease) or Type 2;
- congenital myotonic dystrophy;
- congenital muscular dystrophy;
- one of the congenital myopathies;
- a peripheral neuropathy.

Assessment of hypotonia

This is important to identify the likely anatomical basis of, and therefore the most appropriate approach to, a child with hypotonia, and this may be summarized as follows:

- hypotonia without muscle weakness;
- hypotonia with muscle weakness;

- hypotonia without symptoms/signs suggesting CNS disease;
- hypotonia with symptoms/signs suggesting CNS disease.

History

Important clues as to the likely cause may be obtained from a detailed history, although in isolation, these clues are not necessarily unique to, or pathognomic of, a specific disorder. The history should be thorough.

Antenatally

A maternal history of repeated miscarriages or stillbirths should raise the possibility of a chromosomal or genetic condition, including metabolic disorders.

Polyhydramnios, poor or reduced fetal movements (compared to previous pregnancies), an abnormal fetal lie (i.e. transverse or breech) and a delayed onset of, or failure to undergo, spontaneous labour are frequently found in children with peripheral neuromuscular disorders and less commonly in disorders of the central nervous system.

Pre-term delivery is not specific to any single cause of hypotonia but is more frequently seen in children who have an abnormality of the central nervous system or a genetic/chromosomal disorder.

Birth

Assisted delivery (e.g. forceps or vacuum extraction) and a history of resuscitation are not generally of help in differentiating between the many causes of a floppy infant. However, a newborn infant who requires intensive resuscitation at birth, and who develops early neonatal seizures, is more likely to have a central cause for subsequent hypotonia – either as a result of an hypoxic–ischaemic encephalopathy or due to underlying cerebral dysgenesis.

Perinatal period

A history of respiratory difficulties requiring ventilatory support or feeding difficulties in the absence of an hypoxic–ischaemic encephalopathy, is more commonly found in infants who have either a neuromuscular disorder (e.g. congenital myopathy, congenital myotonic dystrophy or a congenital myasthenic syndrome), a genetic syndrome (e.g. Prader–Willi syndrome) or a metabolic condition (e.g. an organic acidaemia).

Infancy

Persistent respiratory or feeding difficulties in the first few weeks of life would also be more consistent with a neuromuscular cause (e.g. severe spinal muscular atrophy, congenital myotonic dystrophy, a congenital myopathy including myotubular or central core myopathy, or a congenital myasthenic syndrome) or genetic syndrome (specifically, Prader–Willi syndrome). However, swallowing difficulties, often in association with episodes of aspiration may also occur in infants who have a central cause for their hypotonia (e.g. evolving cerebral palsy or the rare 'opercular' or 'perisylvian' syndrome characterized by cerebral dysgenesis in the rolandic or perisylvian region).

A poor cough and reduced spontaneous movements, particularly against gravity (e.g. when being bathed or having a nappy changed) may also indicate a neuromuscular cause. The floppy infant who is also weak usually has an underlying neuromuscular disease.

Delayed development is frequently an associated and important feature. Generally, isolated motor (gross and/or fine) delay would be consistent more with a neuromuscular or, less commonly, a connective tissue disorder, while global developmental delay tends to indicate a disorder of the central nervous system or a chromosomal disorder. However, there are some important exceptions to this rule:

- *Duchenne muscular dystrophy:* although the usual pattern of presentation is with delay in gross motor milestones (specifically, learning to walk independently after 16-18 months of age, an awkward, waddling gait or frequent falls), these boys may present in the first few years of life with global delay, including delayed speech and language, or with poor attention span and behavioural difficulties;
- *Congenital myotonic dystrophy:* these children commonly show global delay (Figure 2.2).

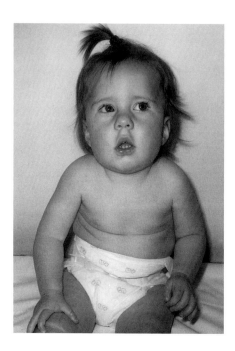

Figure 2.2 *20-month-old infant with congenital myotonic dystrophy.*

Recurrent episodes of transient and self-limiting hypotonia in an otherwise normal infant, **or** exacerbations in a pre-existing hypotonic infant, at times of a febrile illness or other 'stress' (e.g. surgery), should raise the possibility of an underlying metabolic disorder, particularly if they are also sick and acidotic (e.g. Leigh's syndrome, maple syrup urine disease or an organic acidaemia). Acute, though less often marked exacerbations may also be seen in children with neuromuscular conditions including spinal muscular atrophy, congenital muscular dystrophy, a peripheral neuropathy or one of the congenital myasthenic syndromes.

Family history
Parents should be questioned about any personal or family history of any neurological and neuromuscular disorders – specifically myotonic dystrophy and myasthenia gravis – and whether any other children have died in infancy/early childhood. A history of consanguinity should also raise the possibility of a genetically-determined condition, including a metabolic/biochemical disease.

Examination

General physical examination

The general physical examination may give important clues as to the underlying cause of a child's hypotonia.

Reduced facial movement, ptosis and ophthalmoplegia more commonly suggest a neuromuscular cause which may be due to:

- congenital myotonic dystrophy (usually it is the child's mother and not the father who is the affected parent);
- a defect in neuromuscular transmission (e.g. neonatal transient/congenital myasthenia or infant botulism);
- a severe congenital myopathy (e.g. centronuclear [myotubular] myopathy);
- Guillain–Barre syndrome;
- a mitochondrial myopathy;
- infant botulism (these children commonly present between one week and six months of age and usually have a preceding history of constipation followed by profound hypotonia and respiratory distress. Affected infants have dilated pupils that are unreactive to light).

Less commonly, reduced facial movement may be due to a central cause:

- Moebius syndrome caused by dysgenesis/agenesis of brainstem cranial nerve nuclei (Figure 2.3);
- the opercular syndrome (also called the perisylvian or Worster–Drought syndrome) caused by either a congenital or, less commonly, an early acquired abnormality of the opercular or perisylvian region(s);
- the velo-cardio-facial syndrome (associated with a microdeletion of chromosome 22q11.2 identified by Fluorescent In Situ Hybridization or 'FISH') (Figure 2.4).

The presence of abnormal skin pigmentation or texture could indicate the presence of a neurocutaneous disorder (e.g. neurofibromatosis or tuberous sclerosis); however, the characteristic lesions in these conditions may not be obvious or marked in the first year of life. The conjunctival telangiectasias of ataxia-telangiectasia also do not appear until

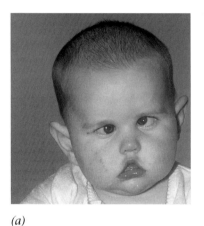 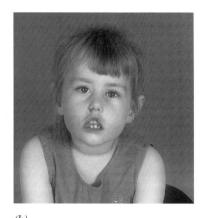

(a)   *(b)*

Figure 2.3 *(a) A six-month-old girl with Moebius syndrome showing marked facial diplegia and also bilateral but incomplete ophthalmoplegia. She showed only minimal global developmental delay. (b) The same girl at 7 years of age trying to smile. Her previous squint had been treated with botulinum toxin injections and surgery.*

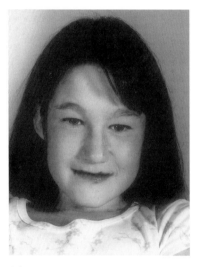 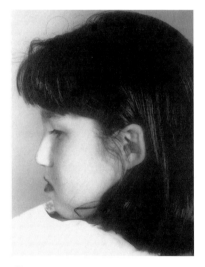

(a)   *(b)*

Figure 2.4 *11-year-old girl with 22q11 deletion. (a) Typical facial features include a wide and prominent root and bridge of the nose with a bulbous tip, hypertelorism with short, narrow palpebral fissures. A small mouth is often characteristic in younger children. (b) The same girl in profile shows a rather square shape to the ears.*

the age of six or seven years, although these children may present in the first few years of life with hypotonia and developmental delay.

Hair appearance and texture may also provide important clues: coarse, dark and excessive hair in the mucopolysaccharidoses; twisted, sparse or 'steely' hair in Menke's syndrome (boys, usually accompanied by severe seizures in infancy) and some organic acidaemias; hair loss/poor hair growth may occur in biotinidase deficiency, arginosuccinate synthetase deficiency and isovaleric acidaemia.

The spine should also be examined for any anomalies (e.g. naevus, lipoma, dimple, hairy tuft/patch), suggesting an underlying spinal dysraphism, and therefore a central or mixed (upper and lower motor neurone) cause of hypotonia.

A bell-shaped or narrow chest and little movement of the chest wall are characteristic features of severe spinal muscular atrophy (Type 1 also called Werdnig–Hoffman disease). They may occasionally be found in a severe congenital myopathy or, less commonly, in a genetic/chromosomal disorder (e.g. the Pena–Shokeir syndrome).

The presence of a cardiomyopathy in the first two years of life should raise the possibility of an underlying metabolic or biochemical disorder (e.g. glycogen storage [Pompe's] disease or a mitochondrial cytopathy). A cardiomyopathy very rarely occurs during infancy with either Duchenne muscular dystrophy or a congenital myopathy but may occasionally be the presenting feature in Friedreich's ataxia.

Hepatosplenomegaly would also be more consistent with a metabolic rather than a peripheral or central cause of hypotonia – including a glycogen storage disorder or a peroxisomal disorder (e.g. Zellweger's syndrome or neonatal adrenoleucodystrophy).

Measurement of the child's current and previous growth parameters (including occipitofrontal head circumference) is important. Microcephaly often reflects an underlying cerebral dysgenesis or an antenatal (e.g. intrauterine infection, maternal substance abuse) or early infantile cerebral insult, sometimes as a sequel to a diffuse hypoxic-ischaemic encephalopathy or meningitis. Macrocephaly should raise the possibility of hydrocephalus, tuberous sclerosis and neurofibromatosis. Macrocephaly may also be found in certain metabolic conditions including glutaric aciduria

Type 1, Canavan's disease, Alexander's disease and untreated congenital hypothyriodism. Although macrocephaly may also be found in children with a neuromuscular cause (e.g. myotonic dystrophy or Duchenne muscular dystrophy), this tends to develop after the age of four or five years.

Multiple joint contractures present at birth may be defined by the term 'arthrogryposis multiplex congenita'. It is important to understand that arthrogryposis is a syndromic and not an aetiologic diagnosis; there are many causes of 'arthrogryposis multiplex congenita' or multiple joint contractures:

- children with severe muscle weakness due to a congenital myopathy, severe congenital muscular dystrophy, congenital myotonic dystrophy, a mitochondrial cytopathy or one of the congenital myasthenic syndromes; contractures present at birth are rarely seen in severe spinal muscular atrophy Type 1 (Werdnig-Hoffman disease);
- children with cerebral or spinal dysgenesis (e.g. lissencephaly or spina bifida);
- children with a chromosomal disorder (e.g. trisomy 8 or 13);
- children whose mothers' pregnancies were complicated by marked oligohydramnios;
- no obvious cause.

Generally, most hypotonic infants with multiple contractures at birth will have a central (CNS) or chromosomal, rather than a peripheral (i.e. neuromuscular) disorder.

Neurological examination

An infant will not usually be able to co-operate with an adult-oriented detailed neurological examination. The approach, and the examiner, should be:

- confident and gentle; the examiner must be prepared to play with the child and appropriate toys (with both the child and the doctor playing on the floor if necessary);
- patient and flexible, making observations as both the child and opportunity allow,

- knowledgeable in basic neuroanatomy so that the question 'where is the lesion' is kept in mind during both the initial observation and subsequent neurological assessment.

Observation

The most important part of the neurological examination is obser-vation – simply watching the child – playing, on their parent's lap, drinking or eating or being undressed, etc . . . This may provide much if not most of the relevant and important information about the child's developmental level and neurological functioning.

A markedly hypotonic infant usually lies in a characteristic posture, often described as 'frog-like' with all four limbs in contact with the surface on which they are lying and with the hips abducted and rotated, the knees slightly flexed and the feet plantar-flexed.

The features to look (and listen) for:

- how alert and responsive is the child;
- does the child appear to see (i.e. fix on and follow visual cues) and hear;
- the child's breathing pattern;
- listen for any vocalization and for the quality of any cry and cough *(an alert infant with a weak cry/cough and poor respiratory movements should raise the possibility of a neuromuscular cause, e.g. from or soon after birth – spinal muscular atrophy, congenital muscular dystrophy, a congenital myopathy or a severe peripheral neuropathy and later in the first year, a myopathy, Guillain–Barre syndrome or a spinal tumour);*
- look for evidence of muscle fasciculation – in the face and fingers/toes as well as the tongue. Gently introducing and withdraw-ing a dummy or the teat of a bottle may be adequate in demonstrat-ing fasciculation. Fasciculation in the fingers and toes is best seen with the child sitting on a parent's lap with the limbs dependent, or by getting the child to reach out for a toy, when the fasciculation may appear more obvious (almost like a low amplitude but 'fast'

tremor). *(Fasciculation in an infant is most commonly found in spinal muscular atrophy [Types 1 or 2] but may be seen in any severe denervating condition, including a peripheral neuropathy).*

Examination

Muscle bulk

An assessment of muscle bulk may also be obtained from inspection but is best obtained from feeling the muscles. In older children muscle wasting may be seen in both central (i.e. CNS) and peripheral (i.e. neuromuscular) conditions – and the pattern of wasting may suggest a myopathy (proximal > distal wasting) or a neuropathy (distal > proximal wasting). However, in the younger child and particularly in the infant, significant muscle wasting is more likely to be caused by a neuromuscular disorder, and one that is often severe in nature.

Muscle strength

One of the most important aspects of the neurological examination when assessing the hypotonic child is muscle strength. **Some doctors consider that hypotonia and muscle weakness are one and the same physical sign; they are not – they are two separate signs.** The presence or absence of muscle weakness is the most important feature in differentiating a central from a peripheral cause for an infant's hypotonia:

- a hypotonic infant who is weak is far more likely to have a peripheral neuromuscular disorder;
- a hypotonic infant who is not weak is far more likely to have a central or chromosomal disorder.

Assessing muscle strength is more difficult in the infant than in the school-age child but must be undertaken to identify any muscle weakness. The weak infant:

- is unable to lift his head against gravity;
- shows little or no resistance to passive stretching of the limbs;
- shows little movement of the limbs when testing primary or automatic reactions (i.e. the Moro reflex, automatic crawling and walking);

- may slip through the examiner's hands when held suspended under the armpits;
- makes little or no attempt to use antigravity muscles when reaching for toys which are held in front or above him.

In the older child (aged four to seven years), the following features are usually associated with muscle weakness:

- the need to hold on to something when trying to stand – particularly when getting up off the floor from a sitting or lying position (called the Gower's manoeuvre);
- the gait is waddling;
- not being able to jump with both feet off the ground;
- the child finds it easier to come down rather than go up stairs.

Muscle stretch reflexes

Muscle stretch (deep tendon) reflexes are frequently given too much importance and are therefore over-interpreted. Reflexes may be more difficult to elicit in infants than in older children. If muscle stretch reflexes are initially difficult to find in older children (>three years), it is useful to repeat with reinforcement. This can be undertaken by having the child squeeze a soft toy or a parent's finger when attempting to elicit reflexes in the legs, and by asking the child to clench the teeth or shut the eyes tightly when attempting to elicit reflexes in the arms. Muscle stretch reflexes that remain absent with reinforcement usually indicate genuine areflexia and is generally pathological. The presence or absence of these reflexes, and whether exaggerated or not, must be taken in conjunction with the overall clinical picture. However, there are some useful generalizations.

- The hypotonic infant who has **brisk** reflexes with or without ankle clonus is more likely to have a central (CNS) condition (e.g. evolving cerebral palsy, often of the dyskinetic type, or an underlying neurodegenerative condition).
- The hypotonic infant who has **absent** reflexes is likely to have

> either severe spinal muscular atrophy (Werdnig–Hoffman disease) or a severe and congenital peripheral neuropathy.
> - The hypotonic infant with **normal** reflexes may have either a peripheral cause (e.g. a mild congenital myopathy, congenital muscular dystrophy, a congenital myasthenic syndrome or an early and mild peripheral neuropathy), a central cause or a genetic disorder.

It must be emphasized that occasionally children may show a combination of signs that suggest both a central and peripheral (neuromuscular) disorder (i.e. hypotonia, muscle weakness and increased muscle stretch reflexes). These include:

- children with a congenital myopathy who, because of premature birth or severe perinatal respiratory difficulties, may also have suffered an hypoxic-ischaemic cerebral insult;
- infants with rare conditions such as metachromatic leucodystrophy, Krabbe's leucodystrophy and biotinidase deficiency;
- spinal abnormality (developmental [dysraphism] or acquired [tumour]).

Parental examination
The child's parents must obviously be asked if they have any neurological symptoms, but it may also be both appropriate and important to *examine* the parents, particularly if a neuromuscular disorder is thought to be the cause of the child's hypotonia. The examiner should assess in each parent:

- the presence or absence of any contractures or pes cavus;
- muscle bulk and strength (including facial muscles and eye closure);
- muscle stretch reflexes;
- presence or absence of myotonia (active or passive).

(Children often find it amusing when their parents are also examined in the clinic and this may even facilitate co-operation with their own examination; only very rarely do children become upset when their parents are examined).

Time course

As with any neurological disorder, observation over time may be very helpful and even provide definitive diagnostic information. This is because of the evolution with time of a number of disorders, during which symptoms or signs or both may become more (or less) obvious. Some of the more common examples include the following.

- The infant with ataxic or dyskinetic cerebral palsy (with predominant cerebellar or basal ganglia involvement, respectively), may initially show only profound hypotonia. The spasticity, dystonic posture and involuntary movements that characterize these syndromes may only become manifest during or after the second or third year of life.
- Hypotonia, often in association with severe feeding difficulties, may be profound in babies/infants with Prader–Willi syndrome, but this becomes less marked and milder (and even subtle) after the age of 18–24 months.
- Progressive disorders may only become apparent with time, and frequently after the first year of life; it is important to ask the child's parents whether their child has lost any skills which could indicate an underlying neurodegenerative disorder.
- Skin lesions in tuberous sclerosis, and particularly in neurofibromatosis, may not become apparent until the second or third year of life, if not later. The conjunctival telangiectasias that characterize ataxia-telangiectasia usually only become apparent after the age of six or seven years.
- Benign congenital hypotonia is firstly uncommon and secondly, being a diagnosis of exclusion, should only be diagnosed *retrospectively*, probably after the first or even the second year of life – by which time the child's tone should have returned to normal. These children should also show normal non-motor developmental milestones.

It is very likely that a number of children previously labelled with 'benign congenital hypotonia' will be found to have an underlying neuromuscular or metabolic disorder, providing they have appropriate evaluation and investigation.

Investigations

As will have been obvious from the range of neurological conditions that may present as a 'floppy' infant, an equally large number of investigations may be required to identify the cause of the hypotonia. The rational approach is to first try and determine whether the child has a central or peripheral (neuromuscular) cause for the hypotonia and also whether the hypotonia could be progressive.

As with any investigation, the more clinical information that can be provided, the better the chance of obtaining a useful result. This is particularly true for neuroimaging, neurophysiology (specifically nerve conduction studies and electromyography), cytogenetics and molecular genetics. If a specific condition, syndrome or chromosomal disorder is suspected, then this should be stated in any request for the relevant investigation(s).

As a general rule, **central** causes are usually investigated by neuroimaging (preferably with magnetic resonance imaging), some biochemical investigations and chromosomal/DNA analysis; **peripheral** neuromuscular causes by measurement of blood creatinine phosphokinase (CPK) levels, nerve conduction studies/electromyography (EMG) and muscle (occasionally, peripheral nerve) biopsy.

- All children with symptoms and signs of the syndrome of cerebral palsy should have brain magnetic resonance imaging (MRI) looking for periventricular leucomalacia, radiological evidence of hypoxic-ischaemic encephalopathy, cerebral or cerebellar dysgenesis or abnormalities of the basal ganglia or deep white matter.
- All children who are weak should have a CPK measurement (markedly elevated in Duchenne/Becker muscular dystrophy [30–100 times normal] but not quite as elevated in the congenital muscular dystrophies, some of the rarer, 'limb-girdle' dystrophies and in some other dystrophies [e.g. myotonic dystrophy, facio-scapulo-humeral dystrophy – 3–10 times normal]). CPK levels are usually normal in the congenital

myopathies, peripheral neuropathies and congenital myasthenic syndromes.

Neurophysiological investigations (nerve conduction studies and EMG) should be able to differentiate a primary muscle disorder (i.e. a myopathy or dystrophy) from a peripheral neuropathy, and may demonstrate a congenital myasthenic syndrome. Muscle biopsy is usually required to identify the specific muscle disease, including differentiating Duchenne and Becker muscular dystrophies.

DNA analysis may also be extremely helpful in diagnosing some of the more common neuromuscular diseases or some of the other hypotonic syndromes:

- Spinal muscular atrophy (Types 1 and 2) – deletion of exons 7 and 8 of the survival motor neuron gene (SMN) gene on chromosome 5q (Figure 2.5);
- Myotonic dystrophy – unstable trinucleotide repeat on chromosome 19 (see Figure 2.2);
- HMSN Type 1a (Charcot Marie Tooth disease) – duplication of the region 17p11.2 or a mutation of the PMP22 myelin protein gene;
- Prader–Willi syndrome – absence of paternal DNA on the chromosome 15q11 locus (Figure 2.6);
- Facio-scapulo-humeral (FSH) dystrophy – most cases linked to a locus on chromosome 4q3.5;
- Rett syndrome – most 'classical' cases (80%) will have mutation of the MECP2 gene on DNA analysis.

Although DNA analysis may be helpful in Duchenne and Becker muscular dystrophy, in the absence of a family history, the deleted or duplicated DNA can rarely differentiate between the more severe, Duchenne and milder, Becker clinical phenotypes. Muscle biopsy can differentiate between the two clinical phenotypes by demonstrating their different abnormal pattern of dystrophin staining.

Blood ammonia and lactate levels, blood and urine amino acids and urine organic acid analyses may suggest a possible underlying metabolic disorder, although usually more detailed investigations, including

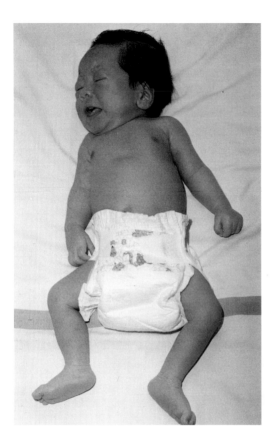

Figure 2.5 Two-month-old infant with severe Type 1 spinal muscular atrophy showing the characteristic 'frog-like' posture with abducted and externally rotated hips and disproportionately normal-looking facies.

skin or muscle biopsies, are required to identify a specific metabolic disorder.

Finally, specialist opinions in paediatric neurology and metabolic disease are important and should be sought in view of the increasing range of identified and specific neuromuscular disorders (e.g. the expanded and still-expanding specific phenotypes in the congenital muscular and limb girdle dystrophies and the congenital myasthenic syndromes) and metabolic disorders (e.g. the mitochondrial cytopathies [including the Leigh's syndrome phenotype], peroxisomal disorders and carbohydrate deficient glycoprotein syndromes).

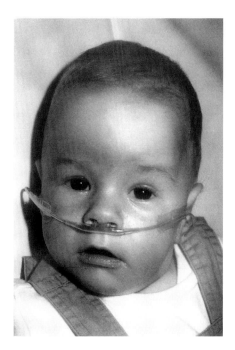

Figure 2.6 *A child with Prader–Willi syndrome.*

Common fallacies

- That the floppy infant cannot have cerebral palsy.
- That muscle stretch reflexes are useful in differentiating a peripheral from a central cause of hypotonia.
- That boys with Duchenne muscular dystrophy only have motor developmental delay and do not have communication and learning difficulties.
- That cerebral palsy is a final diagnosis; there is **always** an underlying cause that must be considered and investigated appropriately.
- That hypotonia is commonly benign and transient and therefore does not need investigating.
- That children do not need to be referred for a paediatric neurological or metabolic opinion.

Further reading

Aicardi J. Diseases of the nervous system in childhood, 2nd edn. London: Mac Keith Press, 1998. pp 697–790.

Dubowitz V. The floppy infant – a practical approach to classification. Dev Med Child Neurol, 1968; 10: 706–10.

Dubowitz V. Muscle disorders in children, 2nd edn. Philadelphia: W.B. Saunders, 1995.

Emery AEH. (ed.) The Muscular Dystrophies. Oxford: Oxford University Press, 2001.

Miller G, Clark GD. The cerebral palsies. Causes, consequences and management. Boston: Butterworth-Heinemann, 1998.

chapter 3

Headache in children

Introduction

- Headache in children is extremely frequent.
- Classification in the (very) young child is often difficult.
- Phenotypic manifestation of various headache types may change with time and age.

Children and parents want:
- to find a cause;
- to obtain pain relief;
- to receive reassurance (e.g. 'there is no brain tumour');
- to know if it will ever resolve ('go away').

The major issues for the paediatrician are:
1. Evaluation of the young child with a headache:
   - no accurate description of pain;
   - not able to localize pain; or
   - 'no pain at all?!'
2. Not missing a brain tumour (or other intracranial disease).
3. Evaluation of the child with non-specific chronic headache who has functional disabilities.

Incidence/prevalence

Headache is a common symptom in paediatric hospital outpatient clinics. Much less is known about the incidence/prevalence and causes of headache in non-hospital populations.

A Dutch study of 1080 schoolchildren, aged 6–16 years, revealed that 46% had experienced headache at least twice in one year. About 10% had experienced two or more headaches in a month, resulting in school absence and interfering with play and sporting activities.

In a population-based study of 2165 children, representing a random sample of 10% of schoolchildren in Scotland aged 5–15 years, the following diagnoses were made:

Type of headache	no (%) of children	estimated prevalence (%)
Migraine	169 (82)	11.3
Tension headache	14 (6.8)	0.9
Specific diagnosis	3 (1.5)	0.2
Non-specific headache	20 (9.7)	1.3
Total	206 (100.0)	

Clinical implications

- Migraine is the most common cause of severe recurrent headache in children, affecting one child in nine between the age of five and 15 years.
- Tension headache is an unusual cause of headache, severe enough to interfere with normal activities.
- Mixed headache syndromes (i.e. migraine and tension headache, migraine and chronic, daily headache) are relatively common in children.
- Other headaches (e.g. symptomatic) are rare, but may still be important in terms of diagnosis and management.

Headache in children: a general approach

		Page
• Clinical evaluation (history, physical examination) ⇓		50–52
• Warning symptoms/signs (symptomatic) type of headache/associated symptoms/ neurological symptoms ⇓	YES ⇒	52–54
NO	YES ⇒	
• Type of headache classifiable? headache with normal examination	migraine (-like)	55–63
	tension type	63–66
⇓		
NO	YES ⇒	
• Non-specific headache. Any clues? (any clue in history whether or not	trauma	67
suggested by parent/child)	epilepsy	68
	(periodic symptoms other than headache)	60–61
⇓		
NO	YES ⇒	
• Non-specific headache, interfering with daily activities	chronic daily headache	63–66
⇓		
NO		
• Non-specific headache, not interfering with daily activities ⇓		

reassurance

(follow-up)

or

re-take the history!

Clinical examination: history, physical examination

Headache history

A clear and detailed account of the features of the headache must be obtained specifically to answer the following three important questions:

- Is the headache a sinister type of headache?
- Can the headache be classified?
- Is the headache interfering with daily activities?

It is important to obtain a detailed account of a typical episode, including the onset and duration of the headache and how the headache ends – spontaneously or only after treatment.

History

occurrence: periodic, episodic, 'attacks', or 'waxing and waning', chronic, daily.

quality: pulsating, throbbing, pounding, pressing ('vice-like'), sharp, stabbing, or constant, dull pressure, heaviness, steady ache, or do not know, unable to describe; more than one type of headache.

location: unilateral, forehead, eye, whole head, back of the head.

intensity: mild or severe and prohibiting or interfering with daily activities; missing school or being sent home from school.

frequency: daily, weekly, monthly.

associated symptoms: *during an episode*: nausea, vomiting, pallor, photophobia, phonophobia, dizziness, vertigo, anorexia, abdominal pain, drowsiness, numbness, paraesthesiae or weakness of any limbs, blurred vision, double vision; *long term*: behavioural change, school failure, anxiety, depression.

duration: of each headache, of symptom free periods; of the entire episode from start to finish (including any aura); change of pre-existing headache (type, severity, frequency).

precipitating ('triggers') or exacerbating factors: disturbed sleep, fatigue, emotional stress, certain foods, minor head trauma, infections; fever; physical activities.

factors that produce relief: sleep, dark room, rest, vomiting, any specific analgesics.

'aura' symptoms: onset, duration, type (see migraine with aura).

family history: migraine; other headache syndromes.

psychosocial history: family; housing conditions; performance and achievement at school; leisure activities and 'life style'; peer group.

medical and/or behavioural disorders in the past/present: developmental problems; previous neurological problems (head injury, meningitis, encephalitis); other problems (ADHD, depression, anxiety disorders); medication (other than headache therapy).

Physical examination

general: alertness, behaviour, 'healthy' or 'ill'; blood pressure, heart rate, temperature; head circumference.

neurological: in the young: skull percussion and/or head tilt; vision, ophthalmoscopy (optic discs, visual fields); pupils and eye movements; movements, power, tone, coordination; speech.

Headache in the young child

suspicion
no localization

episodic change of:
- facial expression
- (type of) crying
- behaviour (agitation, irritability, restlessness, head banging)
- vomiting, pallor relief after sleep (all: non-specific for headache!)

suspicion
localization
(non-verbal communication)

hands on the head

verbalization
poorly (or not) localized
(>2 years)

e.g. 'mama, head';
'boo-hoo, head'
points to side of head

some description of pain;
able to localize
(4 years)
accurate description
(>5–7 years)

> **Headaches in the older child (aged five to 16 years); what children want to know?**
> - What is the cause?
> - What would make it better?
> - The reassurance that they have no life-threatening illness.
> - Will the headaches go away?

Neuroimaging

When should neuroimaging be carried out?

- The rule: suspicion of any type of intracranial pathology (see 'symptomatic headaches').
- The exception: for parental reassurance (only if essential to allow the family to 'move on' and proceed with any management by excluding a serious cause for their child's headache; see also page 65).

MRI or CT scan:

- MRI is superior, in particular for demonstrating posterior fossa and brainstem pathology and an additional advantage is that it does not involve irradiation. Its disadvantages are availability, sedation and cost.
- CT is acceptable in the acute situation, in particular for identifying any haemorrhage, and also as an initial 'screening' investigation to exclude or confirm a cerebral tumour. CT scanning should be undertaken with and without intravenous contrast. The disadvantages are that CT is not ideal in visualizing the posterior fossa, and it involves brain irradiation.

Symptomatic headaches: warning symptoms and signs

Headache and brain tumour:
- increasing frequency and severity (steadily or intermittently);
- on awakening or waking during the night, maximal at onset, improving during the day;

- crying, coughing may increase pain;
- pain relieved by effortless vomiting (without nausea);
- occipital localization (posterior fossa lesion);
- frontal, eye or no specific localization (supratentorial problem or lesion, hydrocephalus).

Associated symptoms:
- drowsiness;
- behavioural change;
- school failure;
- seizures.

Neurological symptoms, with or without localization:
- cracked-pot percussion (in the young infant);
- large head (in the young infant and young child);
- head tilt;
- papilloedema, optic atrophy, visual field deficit (e.g. hemianopia);
- cranial nerve palsies (particularly the 6th or 7th or 4th if there is a head tilt);
- ataxia;
- pyramidal signs.

Headache and brain tumour
- neurological examination: abnormal signs in 90% of children;
- symptoms of raised intracranial pressure;
- symptoms which localize may be absent;
- absence of papilloedema does not exclude raised intracranial pressure.

Headache associated with hydrocephalus:
- in case of hydrocephalus caused by a fossa posterior tumour: see above;
- disproportionately large head (particularly in the young child);
- in arrested hydrocephalus (large head): in case of decompensation after minor trauma or infection and headache: see above;

- with atrial/ventriculoperitoneal shunt: malfunctioning with (severe) headache, visual changes or regression of (school) performance.

Headache and benign (idiopathic) intracranial hypertension:
- headache is the most common presenting symptom;
- also: diplopia (sixth nerve palsy), blurred vision, vomiting;
- optic disc abnormalities (blurred disc margins to gross papilloedema and haemorrhages) in >90% of patients;
- mild ataxia (rarely).

(Sub)acute symptomatic headache:
- infections with fever (most are not serious, e.g. viral, upper respiratory tract);
- more specific infections: sinusitus, meningitis (viral), encephalitis;
- postconcussion;
- postictal (in a child with epilepsy).

Worrying headaches:
- vascular headache, acute and severe (haemorrhage):
  - arteriovenous malformation (sometimes in child known to have epilepsy);
  - aneurysm (subarachnoid or intracerebral, or combined);
  - extra/subdural (acute).
- vascular (non-bleeding):
  - intracranial venous thrombosis (headache, fever, vomiting, altered consciousness) (may resemble acute encephalitis);
  - hypertensive encephalopathy.

In acute vascular headaches, accompanying neurological symptoms such as meningism or focal signs are very common and should justify admission and urgent neuroimaging studies.

Headache and hypertension (hypertensive encephalopathy):
- headache, often episodic;
- altered consciousness;
- tonic–clonic convulsions or, less commonly, partial seizures;
- (causes: autonomic failure, renal failure, phaeochromocytoma).

Migraine

Migraine without aura (previously called common migraine)

The criteria for diagnosing migraine are at least **five** attacks, with:

- unilateral location;
- pulsating quality;
- moderate to severe intensity (interfering with/prohibiting daily activities);
- aggravation by routine physical activity (e.g. walking up stairs);
- attack lasting 2 to 48 hours.

During headache:

- nausea and/or vomiting;
- photophobia and/or phonophobia.

The International Headache Society (IHS) criteria in clinical practice are not sensitive but highly specific, according to expert clinical diagnoses.

The importance of optimal criteria for paediatric migraine without aura
- To establish a definite diagnosis – and therefore enable the use of appropriate, early and effective treatment.
- To differentiate from tension-type headache or other more serious causes of headache.

Although the presence or absence of a positive family history is not used in the IHS diagnostic criteria of migraine (as the family history is often unreliable) it is, however, common practise to consider a positive family history as supporting the diagnosis (in children with migraine, 80% will have a family history of migraine in either a first or second degree relative).

Children with migraine often complain of travel sickness – and this may be the first symptom of migraine in the younger child, before the development of the headache.

In usual clinical practice
- The duration of the headache may be as short as **one hour.**
- Only **one of the following characteristics** is obligatory:
  - unilateral location (low sensitivity, high specificity);
  - pulsating/throbbing quality;
  - moderate to severe intensity.
- Only **one of the following accompanying symptoms** is obligatory:
  - nausea (high sensitivity);
  - vomiting (low sensitivity, high specificity);
  - photophobia;
  - phonophobia (low sensitivity, high specificity).
- Always ask about a **family history of headache (and not just migraine).**

The influence of age on criteria
- Young children (and their parents) may not be able to describe the pain (localization, quality).
- Headache characteristics change and evolve with the child's age (the older the child, the easier to use the formal IHS criteria).

Migraine without aura and/or tension-type headache
Migraine and episodic, tension-type headache (p 63) may co-exist in any child. Key features independent of age are intensity of headache and presence of nausea for migraine and absence of nausea for episodic, tension-type headache. The specific headache syndrome will usually become more obvious with time.

Migraine with aura
This was previously called hemiplegic migraine or migraine accompagnée (using the IHS classification). The criteria are at least two attacks fulfilling (some of) the following:

- one or more fully reversible aura symptoms indicating focal cerebral cortical or brain stem dysfunction:
  - one aura symptom develops gradually over more than 4 minutes, or two or more symptoms occur in succession;
  - duration of aura does not exceed 60 minutes;
  - headache follows the aura with a symptom-free interval of less than 60 minutes (it may also begin before or simultaneously with the aura).

Migraine with aura, in particular migraine with neurological symptoms, is unusual in children but definitely recognisable.

Migraine with hemisyndromes

- more frequent in childhood than in adults;
- attack may be precipitated by minor trauma (heading a ball, blow on the head);
- unilateral symptoms, **but differing sides in different attacks**;
- the hemi-symptoms typically occur as part of the prodrome (followed by severe contralateral headache), although occasionally the first attack may consist of a severe headache, followed by alteration in consciousness and then a progressive hemisyndrome;
- with or without visual symptoms (scintillations or simple scotomata ipsilateral to the side of limb sensory symptoms or paresis);
- unilateral symptoms develop over a period of minutes:
- sensory or motor symptoms in the face, arm, leg;
  - dysarthria and/or dysphasia (irrespective of which side is affected);
  - alteration in consciousness (from confusion to coma).

In children, complications of migraine with hemisyndromes (i.e. cerebral infarction – stroke) are very rare.

Differential diagnosis
In practice this may occasionally be difficult after a first attack, where there is no, or only a mild headache, when the aura always involves the same side or where is no family history of migraine.

- Todd's paresis (epilepsy: post-ictal paresis or weakness suggests far more a diagnosis of epilepsy than migraine);

- vascular disease (e.g. Moya-moya disease);
- metabolic disorder (e.g. mitochondrial cytopathy, homocystinuria).

Investigations in case of doubt

Neuroimaging: possible vascular pathology (CT for acute severe headache to look for evidence of haemorrhage. MRI and MRA to look for evidence of ischaemia, including Moya-moya disease).

EEG: epileptic disorder (benign occipital epilepsy; possible post-ictal Todd's paresis or anomalies of the major cerebral vessels, including Moya-moya disease).

Metabolic screening: urea cycle disorder (ammonia, organic acids); mitochondrial cytopathy including MELAS syndrome (Mitochondrial Encephalopathy Lactic Acidosis and Stroke-like episodes) (lactate).

Basilar migraine (previously called Bickerstaff's migraine)

This follows the general criteria for migraine with aura:

- visual symptoms in both temporal and nasal fields of both eyes;
- dysarthria;
- vertigo;
- tinnitus;
- decreased hearing;
- double vision;
- ataxia;
- bilateral paraesthesiae;
- bilateral paresis;
- decreased level of consciousness.

The constellation of symptoms and signs that constitute the entity of basilar migraine are those that are related to the tissues supplied by the vertebral basilar system, or posterior fossa-related symptoms. These symptoms nearly always precede the headache.

Differential diagnosis

- Posterior fossa pathology;
- Metabolic disorder.

Ophthalmoplegic migraine
- Very rare in children; early age onset;
- when there is prominent periorbital pain, ptosis or pupillary dilatation, then there should be serious consideration of an abnormal blood vessel (either in size or anatomical site) compressing the oculomotor (3rd cranial) nerve, as occurs in other neurovascular compression syndromes including trigeminal neuralgia.

Special variants of migraine
The predominant features are on alteration in consciousness and disordered thought processes:

- Confusional migraine
- 'Alice in Wonderland' syndrome

Confusional migraine
- Rare; usually occurs in children ≥8 years;
- headache often insignificant;
- well known trigger: minor head trauma (occurring 30–60 minutes before the episode);
- confusional symptoms:
  - inattention, distractibility
  - agitation (or even aggressive behaviour)
  - memory disturbance
  - tremulousness, fear
  - duration of 10 minutes to many hours
  - low frequency of attacks (or even a single episode).

Differential diagnosis
A subacute confusional state is **much** more likely caused by:

- drug-induced toxic or metabolic encephalopathy;
- viral encephalitis;
- non-convulsive status epilepticus.

Where there is any doubt about the cause of an acute or subacute confusional state the child should have:

- metabolic (biochemical) investigations (e.g. urea creatinine and electrolytes; glucose; ammonia; lactate; amino and organic acids; porphyrins, etc . . .);
- drug and toxicology screen;
- EEG;
- neuroimaging;
- CSF analysis.

Alice in Wonderland syndrome
(So called because the author Lewis Carroll suffered from migraine.)

- Account of migraine (or positive family history);
- attacks typically as a prodrome;
- perceptual abnormalities:
- complex disorders of auditory and/or visual perception e.g. distortions of body-image, speech or vision;
- apraxia, agnosia;
- déjà vu;
- dreamy, trance-like states;
- the differential diagnosis is as for confusional migraine.

Childhood 'migraine with aura': important considerations
The principal forms of migraine with an obvious aura or significant confusion occurring in childhood should always raise the possibility of an alternative diagnosis – of which there are many.

As usual, a clear and detailed history is important in the diagnostic process.

Migraine equivalents

These are syndromes of migraine without headache. In particular in infants and young infants, paroxysmal or episodic symptomatology may be due to a migraine equivalent based on:

- retrospectively the child develops migraine in later childhood or adult life;
- a positive family history of migraine;
- when the child is able to talk, he/she may describe more typical migrainous headaches.

Benign paroxysmal torticollis of infancy (BPT) and benign paroxysmal vertigo (BPV): see Chapter 1
'Abdominal' migraine

The symptoms are:

- recurrent abdominal (periumbilical) pain that may be severe (normal activities interrupted including absence from school);
- onset three to ten years of age (peak five to nine years), girls more than boys;
- associated with (in order of frequency): pallor, nausea (and/or vomiting), fever, limb pain, migraine headache, and dizziness.

Abdominal migraine should be a diagnosis of exclusion, given the large differential diagnosis of recurrent abdominal pain. A clear association with migraine is unproven. Abdominal migraine **without** a migraine headache is a syndrome of autonomic nervous dysfunction which peaks at five to seven years.

Migraine and epilepsy

At present there is no evidence of a genetic link between migraine and epilepsy. Both conditions are relatively common in childhood and their co-occurrence in any child may simply be coincidental. Rarely one of the channelopathies may cause both migraine and epileptic seizures (e.g. familial hemiplegic migraine – an autosomal dominant calcium channelopathy with the gene defect on chromosome 19p).

Headache is an uncommon, but well recognized accompaniment of epileptic seizures, either in benign occipital epilepsy or during the recovery phase after a tonic–clonic seizure.

The combination of visual symptoms, headache and vomiting in **benign partial epilepsy with occipital paroxysms (BEOP)** may be difficult to distinguish from migraine. In BEOP the following typically occur:

- Seizure semiology may comprise visual symptoms:
  - multi-coloured spots, circles, lines ('phosphenes'), transient scotomas;
  - visual hallucinations (including macropsia, micropsia);
  - hemianopia.
  (The visual symptoms or 'aura' in migraine comprise of straight lines in a zig-zag or fortification pattern and are usually white, silver or gold in colour.)
- Other ictal symptoms:
  - tonic deviation of the eyes (with vomiting) – particularly during sleep;
  - migrainous headache (presenting symptom or simultaneously with other ictal symptoms);
  - autonomic symptoms (nausea, sweating, abdominal pain).
- EEG:
  - occipital paroxysms (spikes or sharp waves, followed by a slow wave).

Therapy of migraine

- It is important to explain what migraine is and to reassure the child and the family that there is no sinister cause for the headache including specifically a 'brain tumour'.
- Try to identify (and eliminate) any obvious provoking or triggering factor. Although triggers are often not found the following may act as triggers:
  - stress and anxiety (particularly in schoolchildren);
  - exercise (with dehydration);
  - tiredness, lack of sleep;
  - dietary factors;
  - in a minority, specific food items or additives frequently precipitate an attack (e.g. cheese, chocolate, coloured sweets, preservatives, caffeine); in general there is no indication for using

strict elimination diets (the usefulness of these diets is not proven);
- irregular life-style, including meals;
- strong light (sunlight).
- Explain the importance of regular sleep, meals and the avoidance of dehydration after exercise.
- Use a headache diary.
- Use a simple analgesic in an **appropriate dose at the earliest symptom** of an attack – including during an aura.
- Prophylaxis is rarely indicated (probably only one in 20 children).

Drug treatment

1 Acute treatment
- During migraine attacks, gastric emptying may be delayed and drug absorption impaired. An anti-emetic drug including domperidone or metoclopramide may be used to improve the absorption and therefore the efficacy of any analgesics.
- Severe vomiting may justify the use of suppositories.
- For children >12 years, sumatriptan nasal spray may prove more effective than any oral preparation.
- Analgesics: paracetamol (acetaminophen), ibuprofen.

2 Prophylactic treatment
- This is usually only prescribed in the following situations: incapacitating attacks not relieved by acute treatment occurring several times per month, over at least three months, and leading to absence from school.
- Medications: propanolol, gabapentin, sodium valproate, pizotifen.

Tension-type headache; daily chronic headache

This was previously called tension headache or stress headache. It has the following characteristics:

- episodic or chronic;
- with or without 'disorder of pericranial muscles';
- the IHS classification of this type of headache is not very practical in paediatrics.

episodic:

- headache lasts from 30 minutes to many days;
- bilateral or affecting the whole head;
- pain may inhibit but not prohibit activities;
- no vomiting, no nausea;
- with or without tenderness of pericranial muscles.

(The sensitivity of these characteristics is good, but the specificity is low.)

chronic:

- daily headache; or
- more than six or seven days per month (for at least three to six months).

The gradual transition from episodic to chronic (daily) headache often prompts referral of the child to the GP or paediatrician. Extensive work-up is usually unhelpful. The basic approach to the child and the family is shown in the box on the next page.

'Tense' or stressful events are often denied by parents or the older child (or both) and therefore the term chronic tension-type headache is not very practical. Chronic or daily headache with no underlying serious cause is often a more acceptable term to parents. In some, but **not all** of these patients, there may be an underlying psychological problem including, rarely, sexual and/or physical abuse. This will need to be carefully assessed in each case and family.

Disturbed sleep patterns may contribute significantly to the occurrence of both episodic and chronic (daily) headache. Causes for disturbed sleep are many and include:

- poor sleep hygiene (no set bed-times, children watching inappropriate TV programmes or videos in bed late into the night, drinking caffeine-containing drinks before going to bed, etc . . .);
- nocturnal hypoventilation (e.g. due to obstructive sleep apnoea) may cause disturbed sleep resulting in headache, nausea and anorexia the following morning.
- nocturnal epilepsy (particularly tonic–clonic seizures).

Some benefit may be obtained from temporary medication (e.g. amitriptyline, melatonin) and improved sleep may result in less frequent headaches.

The child with daily headache

Chronic or daily headache in children may have some migraine-like features, including; unilateral location, nausea, photophobia or even a pulsating character of the pain. The severity of the headache may be quite variable, in both an individual child and between children. There may be a clear discrepancy between 'the incapacitating severity' of the headache and the ability to participate in all daily activities; the 'belle indifference' phenomenon is not uncommon.

Approach

- Parents (and their child) often want a definite explanation or cause for the chronic headache. Normal results of laboratory investigations, neuroimaging studies, or even a more extensive uninformative work-up will not necessarily change this expectation.
- Parents often want reassurance, again, that a brain tumour is not responsible for the headache.
- Parents (usually more than the child), want adequate treatment.

1 Information

If appropriate, it must be explained that focusing only on the cause and the pathogenesis of headache are not particularly important (e.g. 'food allergy', head trauma years ago). Consequently, a single, specific therapy (e.g. 'restrictive diet') is unlikely to be helpful. The importance of any previous normal or negative investigations should also be emphasized. It should be made absolutely clear that, despite negative test results, the child's headache and related problems are being taken seriously.

Additional history may be very important, specifically in the following areas:
- functional disabilities (school absence, no sport activities, etc.);

- life-style, sleep, use of coffee;
- behaviour problems, school phobias, anxieties, even years ago;
- family problems;
- school performance;
- headache syndromes in the family;
- previous and current medications being taken (not just analgesics).

2 Diagnostic and management plan

As the cause of the headache is unknown and investigations have been normal, a specific treatment strategy needs to be offered. This should be a 'two-pronged' approach with both an organic and (neuro) psychological work-up.

Parents are often somewhat reluctant to accept an introduction of a child psychologist or child psychiatrist. It may be helpful to explain your concern about the psychological consequences for the child in being absent from school for any length of time. In addition, formal psychological testing is often required to better understand the child's academic abilities, and particularly identify whether the child may have a specific learning difficulty.

It may be useful to set up an agreement or 'a contract' between parents, the child and the paediatrician – e.g. one week of diagnostic work-up and a second week to start a management plan. In the first week at least some diagnostic tests should be offered. As in the majority of these children the most important investigations have already been done, the physician has to be inventive. This 'two week' approach emphasizes especially the psychological and/or psychiatric inventory of the child and family. After the first week the team meet to discuss the results with parents and child (presenting a diagnosis, i.e. an explanation of the child's headache according to 'the experts'). A management plan can be introduced in the second week. A very strict proposal for follow-up should then be offered. This 'two-pronged approach' has to be worked out according to the specific problems of the individual child; in a few cases admission to the hospital may be necessary.

Post-traumatic headache syndromes

Headache immediately after the head injury

- A diffuse, often throbbing headache developing immediately after, or in the first week following a head injury or whiplash injury is very common.
- Associated symptoms or signs accompanying the headache include: vomiting, nausea, dizziness, lethargy and tiredness.
- In most children the headache resolves after the first few weeks.

There is an unclear and unproven relationship between traumatic brain injury or a whiplash injury and the development of chronic headache; the two are not necessarily directly (i.e. causally) related. Perhaps not surprisingly, a causal relationship is often alleged in litigation cases (e.g. when the child has been involved in a road traffic accident, suffered a head injury and has then developed a frequent, if not daily 'headache').

Miscellaneous

Cluster headache

- This is very rare in children under 10 years of age (usually in teenagers/adolescents).
- Headache is severe, strictly unilateral, (supra)orbital, and/or temporal and lasts 15 minutes to 3 hours.
- It is often associated with one or more of: conjunctival injection, lacrimation, nasal congestion, rhinorrhoea, forehead and facial sweating, miosis, ptosis, eyelid oedema, all occurring on the same side as the headache. The child is often very agitated and distressed.
- Attacks occur in clusters for weeks or months, occurring once every other day to many times a day, separated by remission periods lasting months. Unlike in adults, attacks often occur during the day.
- A video of the attacks may be useful in establishing the diagnosis.

Headache and epilepsy

- Rarely, headache may be the most prominent manifestation of epilepsy and usually only in one epilepsy syndrome – benign partial epilepsy with occipital paroxysms.
- However, post-ictal headaches, in particular after tonic–clonic seizures, are very common.
- See also the section on migraine and epilepsy (pp 61–62).

Common pitfalls

- Not every child who has a headache will have migraine.
- Papilloedema is not invariable in children who have headaches due to raised intracranial pressure.
- In the older child and teenager with a chronic headache, stressful life events may include bullying at school and physical and sexual abuse.

Further reading

Abu-Arafeh I (ed.). Childhood Headache. Clinics in Developmental Medicine 158. Cambridge: Cambridge University Press. 2002. In press.

Abu-Arafeh I, Russell G. Prevalence of headache and migraine in schoolchildren. BMJ 1994; 309: 765–69.

Guidetti V, Galli F. Recent development in paediatric headache. Curr Opin Neurol 2001; 14: 335–40.

Hamäläinen ML. Migraine in children: guidelines for treatment. In: Mallarkey G (ed.). Migraine in perspective. Adis, Auckland, 1999. pp 59–72.

Headache and head injury . . . post hoc, or propter hoc? Editorial. Headache 1988; 28: 228–29.

Hockaday JM, Barlow Ch F. Headache in children. In: Olesen J, Tfelt-Hansen P, Welch KMA (eds). The Headaches. New York: Raven Press, 1993. pp 795–808.

Wöber Ch, Wöber-Bingöl C. Clinical management of young patients presenting with headache. Funct Neurol 2000; 15 (suppl.): 89–105.

chapter 4

The child with learning difficulties

Introduction

The term, 'learning difficulties' in a child implies that the child is of school age and is experiencing difficulties in learning. Learning difficulties in a child are frequently preceded by developmental delay that may or may not have been evident or recognized (and therefore investigated) in the early years of life. Developmental delay (and therefore learning difficulties) is one of the three most common and major problems in paediatric neurology; the other two being cerebral palsy and epilepsy.

> It is also important to appreciate that learning difficulties in a child, irrespective of the cause, may result in secondary behavioural and emotional problems, particularly if the learning difficulties are not recognized early – and appropriately addressed.

The objective of this chapter is to consider the child who has predominantly learning difficulties rather than developmental delay, although there will clearly be areas of overlap and duplication.

The paediatrician, in conjunction with other specialists (specifically paediatric neurology and genetics) has an important role in trying to identify the underlying cause for any learning difficulties, in contributing to the multidisciplinary assessment that may clarify the nature and extent of these difficulties and in the management of any associated medical problems.

The child with learning difficulties may present in many situations:

- the first two to three years of life with global developmental delay or with severe communication difficulties;
- school children when their academic or overall school performance is below average (not meeting expectations) or is causing concern;
- school children with higher order communication and language disorders such as semantic-pragmatic disorders or Asperger's syndrome;
- school children with behavioural problems that have developed secondary to unrecognized specific or global learning difficulties. This is a relatively common presentation of children with attention deficit hyperactivity disorder (ADHD) or disorders of attention, motor and perception (the 'DAMP' syndrome).

Learning disability or difficulty replaces the labels mental (or intellectual) retardation and mental handicap. A pragmatic classification that is based simply on the intelligence quotient (IQ) is:

- severe (IQ <50; 'educationally subnormal [severe]', ESN(S) children);
- mild or moderate (IQ 50–70; 'educationally subnormal [moderate]', ESN(M) children);
- borderline (IQ 71–84).

(However, it is of more practical benefit to understand the specific type or nature of any learning difficulties rather than simply the overall total IQ score).

Developmental delay or learning difficulties may be recognized early or late depending on the severity of the problem and whether the child has any other signs including dysmorphic features, neurological abnormalities or other medical problems. The perception and expectations of the child's parents, the presence or absence of siblings and the awareness of health care and educational professionals may also influence the age at which these difficulties are identified – as well as their subsequent management.

Assessment

History

It must be emphasized that the history must be detailed and should cover the pregnancy, delivery and the perinatal period, family history (specifically qualifications achieved by the child's parents, their occupations and a history of learning difficulties or neurological disease in other family members), drug and past medical histories.

The following specific questions must be addressed when faced with a child with developmental delay or learning difficulties:

- Are the learning difficulties isolated with no other neurological symptoms/problems?
- Are the learning difficulties global or specific?

  It is clearly very important to identify whether the child may have a very specific problem such as deafness or blindness.

  Global developmental delay or learning difficulties imply a generalized impairment of cognitive (intellectual) functioning, while specific learning difficulties only involve certain specific intellectual skills. Any standardized intellectual assessment should attempt to differentiate between the child with global and specific learning difficulties. This requires significant expertise and is easier to undertake in the school, rather than the pre-school child. However, a child's pattern of play may provide important early clues and comments from the child's playgroup or nursery staff may be very helpful.

  Language is the most sensitive indicator of overall developmental status and is usually highly predictive of early school success – or failure.

- Is the problem of recent onset or long-standing (specifically from, or soon after birth)?

  Reference to the child's pre-school and school child health surveillance records may help to not only clarify whether any problems are recent or long-standing, but also provide information on the evolving patterns or types of any difficulties.

- Is the problem static (non-progressive) or progressive?

  The vast majority of children with developmental delay or learning difficulties will have a static and non-progressive course.

At the initial consultation it may be difficult to determine whether a child's developmental delay or learning difficulties are static or progressive. It may therefore be necessary to monitor the child for a period of time before this becomes clear. It must also be appreciated that a child may change but not actually deteriorate with time, even though they do not have an underlying progressive disorder. It is also important to understand that a child whose school performance appears to be declining may simply have reached a plateau or is showing a significantly slower than average progress in their academic abilities, is unable to 'keep up' and is therefore falling further away from their peers. Figure 4.1 demonstrates the importance of follow-up and monitoring over time of a child who presents at any given age with developmental delay.

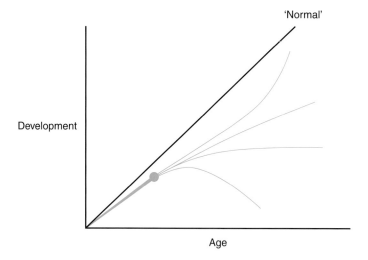

Figure 4.1 *Importance of follow-up of a child who presents at a given age (●) with 'developmental delay'.*

- Could the child have 'pseudo-retardation' or 'pseudo-dementia'? This is a phenomenon that may be seen in a number of situations:

- in children who are emotionally (and physically) deprived;
- in children who have severe and/or chronic medical illnesses necessitating prolonged hospitalization;
- in children who have significant visual or hearing difficulties (particularly if these are not detected early);
- in children with epilepsy (which may reflect transient cognitive impairment, due to either very frequent seizures or the somewhat controversial phenomenon of 'sub-clinical epileptiform activity', including electrical or non-convulsive status epilepticus or continuous spike wave in slow sleep – called CSWSS, or any drugs that are used to treat the epilepsy, particularly if more than two drugs are used and/or in high doses.)
- Could the cause be potentially treatable (i.e. reversible)?
- Is it familial?
- Does the child have abnormal physical findings?
  - general examination (e.g. dysmorphism, micro or macrocephaly or a neurocutaneous syndrome);
  - neurological examination (e.g. hemiplegia, diplegia, ataxia).

Wherever possible, parents should be asked for their permission for the doctor to contact the child's playgroup, nursery, primary or secondary school for information on the child's:

- academic performance;
- physical (games and sports) abilities;
- behaviour (ability to mix with their peers, socialize and their relationship with other children and teaching staff).

Examination

All children must be examined carefully, looking for evidence of a genetic (including chromosomal) syndrome or accompanying neurological signs:

- height (length), weight and head circumference (and relevant centile charts with previous measurements); palmar and plantar skin creases;

- abnormal cutaneous pigmentation or texture, including abnormal fat distribution;
- presence or absence of hepatosplenomegaly;
- presence or absence of any cardiac abnormalities;
- abnormal patterns of behaviour, including repetitive stereotypies (hand-flapping or wringing, body hugging, hyperventilation, autistic features);
- sensory examination, specifically, eyes [vision] and ears [hearing];
  (If the child has visual impairment, is this due to an error in refraction, an optic nerve or a retinal abnormality or a cortical problem. If there is any hearing impairment, is it sensorineural or conductive in origin. This information may provide clues as to the cause of the child's learning difficulties).
- examination of the optic fundi may reveal important diagnostic clues: (e.g. phakomata [tuberous sclerosis], abnormal retinal pigmentation [congenital infections and metabolic disorders, specifically peroxisomal disorders], optic nerve hypoplasia [septo-optic dysplasia], cherry red spot [Tay-Sachs disease and other metabolic disorders]).
- neurological examination;
- parental head circumferences should also be measured if the child has either a small or large head.

The child's development must also be assessed; for children aged two years and under a Denver Developmental assessment may be adequate but for older children, more formal and standardized testing should be used with the specific assessment dependent on local expertise and preference (e.g. Bayley, Griffith's, WISC(R)). Denver testing may not identify mild developmental delay.

In many situations it would be appropriate to obtain formal speech and language, occupational, physiotherapy and educational psychology assessments – as part of the multidisciplinary approach to these children. This is particularly important for children who are considered to have a specific communication problem including semantic-pragmatic language disorder, autism and Asperger's syndrome.

Aetiology

The identification of a specific cause is considerably higher in those children who have **regression** and a **progressive course** to their developmental delay or learning difficulties. Approximately 50% of children with static, non-progressive learning difficulties will be found to have a specific cause – which clearly means that 50% will not be found to have a specific cause, despite extensive investigation.

A cause will be found in approximately 80% of children with severe learning difficulties, 30% of children with mild or moderate learning difficulties and 10% or less of children with borderline learning difficulties. The most common causes of all learning difficulties (irrespective of degree) include:

- a sequel of perinatal hypoxic-ischaemic encephalopathy;
- a sequel of prematurity/extreme prematurity;
- cerebral dysgenesis;
- a fetopathy (e.g. fetal exposure to alcohol, prescribed and recreational drugs);
- chromosomal and genetic disorders.

The aetiology of developmental delay and learning difficulties may be classified generally into prenatal, perinatal, postnatal and uncertain causes. Generally, prenatal conditions are responsible for approximately 60% of causes in children with severe, and 25% of causes in children with mild or moderate learning difficulties.

Learning difficulties of perinatal origin are very rarely isolated but are usually accompanied by cerebral palsy or epilepsy, or both.

The following general classification indicates the time of **origin** of the causes of learning difficulties, but not necessarily when they **present**. A number of these disorders and the accompanying learning difficulties may not become apparent until much later – specifically many of the metabolic disorders.

Prenatal

- Chromosomal disorders (e.g. trisomies, Fragile X)
- Genetic syndromes (e.g. Rett, Angelman syndromes)
- Cerebral dysgenesis (brain malformations including tuberous sclerosis, neurofibromatosis and lissencephaly)
- Familial (parental learning difficulties)
- Drug and toxin exposure (e.g. alcohol, anti-epileptic drugs [phenobarbitone, phenytoin, sodium valproate])
- Intrauterine/congenital infections (including HIV)

Perinatal

- Perinatal hypoxic-ischaemic encephalopathy
- Periventricular haemorrhage
- Birth trauma
- Neonatal hypoglycaemia and hyperbilirubinaemia
- Metabolic disorders (e.g. mitochondrial or peroxisomal disorders)

Postnatal

- Infections of the CNS (meningitis and encephalitis)
- Traumatic brain injury (accidental and non-accidental)
- Non-traumatic brain injury (e.g. hypoxic insults following cardiac arrest or drowning)
- Cultural (e.g. under-stimulation, emotional and physical deprivation)
- Metabolic disorders (e.g. aminoacidopathies, hypothyroidism, mitochondrial or peroxisomal disorders, leucodystrophies, mucopolysaccharidoses)
- Epilepsy (either the epilepsy syndrome itself [e.g. frequent epileptic discharges in the malignant epilepsy syndromes, non-convulsive status epilepticus], or the underlying cause or, occasionally, its treatment)

Uncertain

- Autism and Asperger's syndrome

Investigation

Identifying a cause for a child's learning difficulties is important for many reasons:

- To provide an answer or explanation for the child's difficulties – this is particularly important for parents to know 'why' their child has learning (and other) difficulties.

(However, it is important not to focus exclusively on establishing a diagnosis without actually understanding and addressing the child's difficulties and needs – for many reasons. Firstly, it may not be possible to establish a diagnosis and secondly the child's specific difficulties should be addressed in their own right irrespective of whether any unifying diagnosis is identified – and this is important for both the family and all professionals involved with the child).

- To provide a prognosis regarding developmental outcome and give realistic educational and employment expectations.
- For genetic implications (recurrence risks; risks to the offspring of the affected child).
- For potential and specific therapeutic implications (although this is rarely feasible).
- To identify the most relevant professional and voluntary support groups/associations for the family.

The investigation of children with developmental delay or a learning difficulty should not be based on either an 'all or nothing' or 'screening' principle but on a rational and directed approach based on a detailed history and examination. The approach to the child who has a clear history of progressive difficulties and in whom certain skills or abilities may have been lost (i.e. regression) and who is still deteriorating is quite different from the child whose learning difficulties have been present for some years and are not deteriorating.

The child who appears to have a progressive neurological disorder should be referred for a paediatric neurology opinion.

Additional assessments (speech and language; occupational; physiotherapy; educational psychology)

Additional detailed assessments by therapists, particularly occupational and speech/language and also by psychologists, may provide invaluable information, with regard to both providing an explanation (although not necessarily a specific cause) for the child's difficulties and advising on an appropriate management programme. These assessments should be used in conjunction with relevant investigations.

Specific areas where these assessments may be extremely useful include:

- DAMP syndrome (Deficits in Attention, Motor skills and Perception – also sometimes called, rather inappropriately, 'dyspraxia' or 'the clumsy child syndrome'): these children often have balance and co-ordination, visuo-spatial and concentration/attentional problems. They may also simply present as being 'hyperactive'.
- Asperger's syndrome: incidence of approximately 1 in 5000; motor co-ordination problems, delay in expressive speech, repetitive play, little or no gestures or facial expression, lack of feelings for others and insensitivity (often very marked) to social cues, varying degrees of solitariness or isolation, and specific areas of above average 'intelligence' leading to all-absorbing and even eccentric interests. Severe learning difficulties are uncommon. (Autism and semantic-pragmatic language disorder show similar, overlapping features).
- Autism: often (but not always) 'normal' to the age of 15 or 18 months followed by loss of any acquired language and subsequently, grossly delayed communication skills; avoidance of eye contact, marked withdrawal and a severe impairment of interpersonal relationships; IQ <70 in 70–80% of children; frequent stereotyped, repetitive and obsessional behaviour and an intense dislike of change in their environment. Increased incidence of epilepsy (but **not** increased in Asperger's syndrome).

Neuroimaging

MRI, in preference to CT should be undertaken in **every** child who has evidence of developmental/cognitive regression.

MRI, again in preference to CT, should be undertaken in the child with developmental delay or learning difficulties that is either static or progressive and who **in addition also** has:

- micro- or macrocephaly;
- unexplained dysmorphic features, particularly if suggesting a midline abnormality (e.g. hypertelorism);
- abnormalities of skin pigmentation or texture (e.g. possible tuberous sclerosis, neurofibromatosis or ataxia-telangiectasia);
- abnormal neurological signs (e.g. diplegia, hemiplegia, ataxia, chorea, athetosis);
- epilepsy (particularly if infantile spasms, myoclonic, tonic or focal [partial] seizures);
- significant visual difficulties (of either anterior visual, or cortical origin).

MRI is preferable to CT because it better demonstrates cerebral dysgenesis and specifically abnormalities of neuronal migration and gyration. However, MRI may not definitively identify an underlying leucodystrophy until the age of two to three years when myelination is near completion. CT is often better at demonstrating intracranial calcification.

Other imaging

Other radiological investigations will be determined by the individual child.

- Skull X-ray: there is almost no indication for this procedure. Although it may be helpful in craniosynosotosis, or intrauterine/congenital infections, MRI or CT usually provide evidence of either as well as additional and usually diagnostic information.
- Spine X-rays: of limited use other than in the mucopolysaccharidoses or in Aicardi syndrome (both showing abnormalities of the vertebral bodies).

- Long bones: occasionally these may provide radiological evidence of a peroxisomal disorder (epiphyseal stippling).
- Wrist: bone age estimation may be helpful in assessing bone age in some of the genetic or endocrine syndromes featuring abnormalities of body size/weight (e.g. Sotos syndrome, Figure 4.2).

Cytogenetic testing

Cytogenetic and/or molecular genetic testing should be undertaken if the child shows any dysmorphic features or if there is a family history of similar problems or possible inherited disorders, particularly if there is consanguinity.

It is important to realize that a standard 'karyotype' analysis examines only major chromosome abnormalities. A request for chromosomal analysis should be accompanied by full clinical details including physical and neurological findings and the family history. If a specific syndrome is suspected, or needs to be confirmed or excluded, this should be clearly stated.

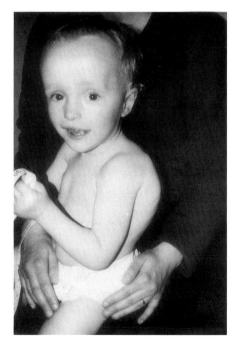

Figure 4.2 Two-and-a-half-year-old child with Sotos syndrome.

Conditions which feature moderate or severe learning difficulties and which are not uncommonly overlooked or not considered, and which may be identified by DNA analysis include the following:

- Fragile X (Xq27.3): 1 in 2000–3000 males, normal body growth and normal or excessive head growth, long face with prominent jaw and/or ears, macro-orchidism, hyperextensible skin and joints, autistic features, epilepsy (the facial and other somatic features may be easier to recognize after puberty). It would be reasonable to undertake Fragile X analysis in any boy with autism. Some female carriers may also have learning difficulties. Fragile X should be undertaken in boys and girls with unexplained learning difficulties particularly if there is a clear family history of learning difficulties.
- Angelman syndrome (maternally-derived deletion on chromosome 15q11–13): age at diagnosis one to four years, global developmental delay with severe communication problems, epilepsy, happy disposition and a paroxysmal, infectious laugh, characteristic facies (Figure 4.3).

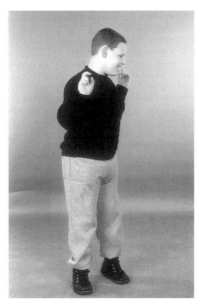 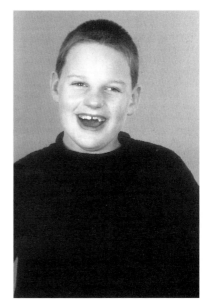

Figure 4.3 *12-year-old boy with Angelman syndrome*

- Rett syndrome (chromosome Xq28; MECP2 mutation): 1 in 10 000–15 000 girls, age at diagnosis 6–18 months, loss of hand function with stereotyped hand movements including 'wringing' or washing movements, acquired microcephaly, epilepsy (with often very characteristic EEG features), autistic features, scoliosis. The common mutation is found in approximately 80% of girls. (The clinical phenotype of 'Rett syndrome' is becoming increasingly wider and the 'classical' phenotype with the MECP2 mutation has also been identified in boys).
- Prader–Willi syndrome (paternally-derived deletion on chromosome 15q11–13): marked feeding difficulties and often profound hypotonia in the neonatal period/early infancy, hip dislocation (10%), mild to moderate developmental delay (motor and social > speech and language), small hands and feet, hypogenitalism, hyperphagia, obesity and short stature from two to three years of age onwards.
- Duchenne muscular dystrophy: a CPK should be measured in all boys under the age of two/three years with unexplained developmental delay, particularly if independent walking was achieved after the age of 18 months and/or if there were early communication problems. The CPK is usually elevated to 30–100 times normal. A deletion or duplication of DNA will be found in approximately 66% of affected boys.
- Williams syndrome (chromosome 7): feeding difficulties, hypercalcaemia/hypercalciuria, elfin facies with wide mouth, aortic/pulmonary stenosis, behaviour problems (solitary, irritable, sleep and anxiety problems, over-friendly with strangers) (Figure 4.4).
- Myotonic dystrophy (chromosome 19): although presentation is usually at birth, with marked hypotonia and weakness (when the child's mother is usually the affected parent), presentation may be in the first or second decade with either muscle symptoms and/or mild or moderate learning difficulties (children presenting outside the neonatal period are often misdiagnosed as simply being poor at sports, having co-ordination problems or being 'dyspraxic') (Figure 4.5a, b).
- Smith–Magenis syndrome (chromosome 17p): incidence is thought to be at least 1 in 25 000 births and children usually present with

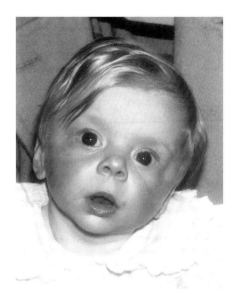

Figure 4.4 *Nine-month-old girl with the typical facial features of Williams syndrome, who presented with delayed motor development and hypotonia and was found to have hypercalcaemia and supravalvular aortic stenosis. Chromosome 'FISH' studies demonstrated an elastin deletion.*

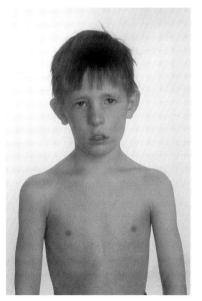

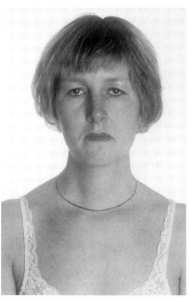

(a)   (b)

Figure 4.5 *(a) Nine-year-old boy and (b) his mother, both affected with myotonic dystrophy. (The child's mother was diagnosed after the disorder was diagnosed in her son at seven years of age.)*

moderate or severe global developmental delay and subsequently learning difficulties. Behavioural problems are common and include self-
injury (with head banging, hand-biting, picking the skin around finger
nails and nail-tearing); body-hugging is also common. There are characteristic facial features (Figure 4.6) and the children are of short stature.

The child should be referred to a clinical geneticist if there is a dis-
tinct possibility that the child may have a chromosomal or genetic
disorder or syndrome.

Metabolic/biochemical investigation

The list of metabolic disorders that may present with, or feature
developmental delay/learning difficulties is extensive. There is no jus-
tification for subjecting these children to all possible metabolic investigations – this is not cost-effective and subjects the child to
unnecessary and often invasive procedures. Similarly, the yield from
undertaking a number of 'routine' or 'screening' investigations (other
than thyroid function) is low and also cannot be justified.

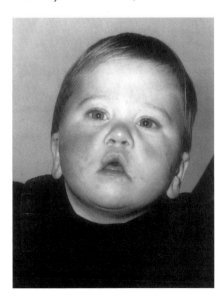

*Figure 4.6 21-month-old boy
with Smith–Magenis syndrome,
who presented with developmental delay and poor growth. He
shows midfacial hypoplasia,
anteverted nares, a tented upper
lip and small hands and feet.
Behavioural problems (including
head-banging) developed from
two years of age. Chromosome
'FISH' studies revealed 17p deletion.*

The rational approach is to undertake only those investigations that appear to be most relevant depending on the child's history and examination. In general, the chance of identifying a metabolic disorder is considerably higher if a child shows evidence of the following:

- other medical problems (specifically feeding difficulties, recurrent vomiting or failure to thrive);
- intermittent episodes of profound lethargy and drowsiness with or without seizures and with or without an abnormal respiratory pattern in association with relatively mild or trivial intercurrent illnesses (e.g. Leigh's syndrome);
- regression (because most of the progressive, neurodegenerative diseases tend to have a metabolic or biochemical basis);
- Lesch–Nyhan syndrome: a serum uric acid should be measured in all boys who present in the first two years of life with unexplained, usually severe, developmental delay, involuntary movements and self-mutilation in the absence of any known perinatal event or insult. The serum uric acid is usually markedly raised in children with Lesch–Nyhan syndrome. There are milder variants when the serum uric acid may be within normal limits and the diagnosis may then be established by demonstrating a deficiency or absence of hypoxanthine-guanine phophoribosyltransferase (HGPRT);
- Adrenoleucodystrophy: blood very long chain fatty acids should be measured in any boy who presents between four and 12 years of age with a decline in school performance, epilepsy, visual difficulties and/or ataxia;

Generally, learning difficulties, dementia and behavioural (including neuro-psychiatric) problems are characteristic presenting features in children aged five to 15 years in the following conditions:

- A leucodystrophy – specifically, adrenoleucodystrophy (accompanied by visual failure, ataxia and epilepsy), juvenile metachromatic leucodystrophy (accompanied by a spastic/dyskinetic gait, ataxia and, later, by areflexia), juvenile Krabbe's disease (rarely seen and accompanied by spinocerebellar degeneration) and juvenile Niemann–Pick disease Type C (accompanied by oculomotor abnormalities, specifically loss of vertical upgaze and ataxia).

- Juvenile neuronal ceroid lipofuscinosis (usually preceded by visual failure and seizures and subsequently the development of extrapyramidal and cerebellar signs).
- Subacute sclerosing panencephalitis (SSPE; usually accompanied by myoclonic and tonic–clonic seizures).
- Wilson's disease (accompanied by facial and limb dystonia, drooling and involuntary movements).
- Juvenile Huntington's disease (father invariably affected; usually accompanied by intractable seizures and rigidity which precedes the development of involuntary movements).
- Variant CJD (initial psychiatric symptoms and cognitive decline at 11–14 years of age followed by visual symptoms, persistent painful sensory symptoms in limbs, ataxia and other abnormal movements and eventually by akinetic mutism).

All children who are thought to have a metabolic problem should be referred for a paediatric neurological or metabolic opinion.

Electroencephalography

The role of the EEG generally, and particularly in children with developmental delay or learning difficulties, with or without behavioural problems, is often over-emphasized and also misinterpreted. The EEG is important in classifying a specific epilepsy syndrome and may also provide important clues to the underlying aetiology of a child's epilepsy.

In the context of the child with developmental delay or learning difficulties, particularly if the child also has acquired communication difficulties, a baseline waking and/or sleeping or 24-hour EEG should be undertaken in the following situations:

- All children with developmental delay or learning difficulties that are considered to be progressive in nature, whether or not they have epilepsy. In the child who has epilepsy, the EEG may provide evidence for a single, unifying cause for the delay and epilepsy (e.g. Angelman and Rett syndromes, late infantile neuronal ceroid lipofuscinosis).

- Children with epilepsy who are showing evidence of either cognitive decline or the development of neurological signs (specifically ataxia); it is frequently assumed that these difficulties are related to either frequent seizures or the effects of anti-epileptic medication, or both. An underlying neurodegenerative cause should always be considered in these children (e.g. cognitive decline, loss of hand and other function and ataxia in children with myoclonic epilepsy aged three to five years should raise the possibility of late infantile neuronal ceroid lipofuscinosis and in older children, subacute sclerosing panencephalitis [SSPE] or one of the other progressive myoclonic epilepsies).

- All children who develop an **acquired** speech and language difficulty that is either receptive and/or expressive in nature. This includes children with autism and in children considered to have the Landau-Kleffner syndrome or the syndrome of electrical status epilepticus of slow-wave sleep ('ESESS') which is also called continuous spike wave in slow sleep ('CSWSS').

- All children with epilepsy and learning difficulties who are said to have repeated and often prolonged (usually hours or even days) periods of 'switching-off', being 'too quiet' or 'not speaking normally' – to exclude episodes of electrical or non-convulsive status epilepticus (the child's parents and teachers should be particularly listened to in this specific situation – they know their child best!).

Specialist opinion

The degree of investigation of the child with learning difficulties will depend on the individual child and the level of suspicion of an underlying cause (and what that cause might be), the experience of the paediatrician and the availability of resources and specifically the availability of specialist investigations.

A child with learning difficulties should be referred to and assessed by a specialist in neurological, metabolic or clinical genetics in the following situations:

- the child who appears to have a progressive neurological disorder;
- the child who has no identified cause for the learning difficulties;
- the child with epilepsy in whom the seizures are poorly-controlled or who may be experiencing episodes of non-convulsive status epilepticus or periods of transient cognitive impairment, or both;
- the child who may have a possible metabolic disorder;
- the child who appears to have a chromosomal or genetic syndrome.

Management

As already stated, the paediatrician has a key role in helping to recognize the child with learning difficulties and in identifying an underlying cause for these difficulties.

An interdisciplinary approach is essential for a number of reasons:

- in diagnosing the type, extent and where possible the cause of the learning difficulties;
- in implementing an appropriate management programme;
- in regularly reviewing the child's medical, therapy and educational needs; certain metabolic disorders or genetic/chromosomal syndromes may take time to evolve and the child's (and the family's) needs may understandably change over time;
- in identifying appropriate professional support for the child and family (this may involve psychology, child psychiatry, social work and the provision of short-term respite care);
- in planning for the child's future;
- in ensuring good communication and liaison with the child's parents and all professionals involved with the family – particularly in primary care and the community;

- in trying to ensure that the child is placed in the most appropriate school for their physical and educational needs;
- in being aware of the relevant legislation and identifying all the available state and private welfare benefits for which the child and the family may be eligible;
- in providing the family with the names, addresses, telephone numbers and web-site addresses of the relevant voluntary support and other organizations.

In the pre-school child the paediatrician is likely to be the most appropriate professional to co-ordinate this interdisciplinary process. In the school child, this role is probably more appropriately undertaken by teaching staff although the community paediatrician and school doctors continue to have an important role and function.

There are a number of medical problems that occur more commonly in children with learning difficulties, particularly when the difficulties are severe. These should be anticipated wherever possible and include the following:

- epilepsy;
- spasticity (and contractures);
- feeding difficulties and constipation;
- sleep impairment (a very important issue, particularly for the family);
- chest infections with or without episodes of aspiration;
- behavioural difficulties;
- stress-related illnesses in the parents and siblings (which may result in additional and major psychological and family dynamic difficulties, including unemployment, divorce, depression and suicide).

The successful management of all of these problems will usually require specialist advice. Again, it is important that the problems are identified and addressed as early as possible.

Common fallacies

- that most children with learning difficulties are unlikely to have an underlying cause;
- that boys with some primary muscle disorders including Duchenne muscular dystrophy or myotonic dystrophy do not have non-motor developmental delay or learning difficulties;
- that learning difficulties in a child with epilepsy are usually due to the epilepsy or its treatment with anti-epileptic drugs; any learning difficulties are more typically caused by the underlying aetiology of the epilepsy (whether this aetiology is identified or not);
- that children with cerebral palsy always have learning difficulties;
- that children with learning difficulties do not require investigation;
- that children with learning difficulties do not necessarily need to be referred for a paediatric neurological or clinical genetics opinion;
- that communication between hospital and community child health services and between child health and education services is usually adequate.

Further reading

Curry CJ, Stevenson RE, Aughton D et al. Evaluation of mental retardation: recommendations of a consensus conference. Am J Med Genet 1997; 72: 468–77.

Gordon N. Specific learning disorders: motor skills, language and behaviour. In: Brett EM (ed.). Paediatric Neurology, 3rd edn. Edinburgh: Churchill Livingstone, 1997. pp 455–76.

Wilska ML, Kaski M. Why and how to assess the aetiological diagnosis of children with intellectual disability/mental retardation and other neurodevelopmental disorders: description of the Finnish approach. Euro J Paediatr Neurol 2001; 5: 7–13.

Index